D1458546

Miraculous Breakthroughs
For Prostate and
Impotency Problems

**Miraculous Breakthroughs for
Prostate and Impotency Problems**

A Practical Guide to Prostate Health

FISCHER PUBLISHING CORPORATION
Canfield, Ohio 44406

Miraculous Breakthroughs For Prostate and Impotency Problems

Advice On
Prevention • Self-Treatment
Medication • Testing

William L. Fischer

Fischer Publishing Corporation
Canfield, Ohio 44406

Disclaimer

This book is informational only and is not intended as a substitute for consultation with a duly-licensed medical doctor. Any attempt to diagnose and treat illness should come under the direction of a physician. This author is not a medical doctor, and does not purport to offer medical advice, make diagnoses, prescribe remedies for specific medical conditions or substitute for medical consultation.

Nothing noted in the text should be considered an attempt by William L. Fischer or the publisher to practice medicine, prescribe remedies, make diagnoses or act as persuasion for enforcing some mode of surgery. Instead, knowledge received is strictly for purposes of education. William L. Fischer takes no responsibility for its content.

Table of Contents

Preface

Dear Friends:

Prostate disorders of some form, statistics tell us, will affect the average man over age 40 sometime during his life. One in 11 white men, moreover, will develop prostate cancer this year - and one in 9 black men will. Pretty scary facts.

But these figures aren't etched in stone. The average man can reduce his chances of developing prostate cancer and other prostate problems with some simple, common sense steps.

This is the objective of this book - to help men prevent prostate problems and cancer. For those who are quietly suffering with these conditions, the goal is to find ways to relieve the pain.

The reader will find diagnostic and treatment methods used by modern medicine outlined here, as well as several prostate relievers and cures that lie outside the medical mainstream.

Nutritional research is finding that the key to a lifetime free of prostate troubles is lying on your dinner plate - or should be. A proper diet, plus several nutritional supplements, can help men avoid and alleviate prostate ailments.

Exercise is also an important part of keeping the gland free of prostatitis or prostatic hypertrophy well into a man's golden years. This updated and fully revised edition of *Miraculous Breakthroughs* explains which exercises are the best, and why. In fact, this book provides invaluable insight into natural ways of staying healthy and having prostate problems solved before they manifest themselves.

The same prescription applies to men who want to avoid prostate cancer. I have included instructions for an important self-examination for detecting testicular cancer. It is not a widely known disease, but it is deadly if not discovered in time.

The delicate subject of impotency is examined with honesty and sensitivity, in language easy for the layman to understand. It offers hope through natural methods as well as new remedies only recently obtainable in the United States.

This book deserves the attention of every man - and of any woman concerned about the well-being of her male loved-ones. It de-mystifies the prostate gland and provides hope to those who suffer from impotency. It is hoped that this updated edition of *Miraculous Breakthroughs for Prostate and Impotency Problems* will be a friend wherever it goes; that it will help you to return to nature's way of caring for your body.

William L. Fischer, publisher

Comments and Reviews
for "Miraculous Breakthroughs for Prostate and Impotency Problems;" first edition.

John Orsini,
athletic trainer, UCLA
former National Weightlifting Champion:

"As a sports figure and health expert, I found William Fischer's book *Miraculous Breakthroughs* to be a jewel. Not only did I find the advice concerning the prostate gland and impotency to be sound, I recommended the book to several of my friends. These older gentlemen were all suffering from some type of prostate problem.

They were relieved to read a book which understood their pain, and were delighted when they put the advice into practice. Between the natural products, such as Flower Pollen Extract and Kombucha, and the dietary guidelines (important for every man to read, regardless of his age or the state of his prostate), each of my friends found a method or combination of methods which alleviated his problem. None of them suffer any longer - thanks to William Fischer's *Miraculous Breakthroughs.*

This may just be the most important book you read this year. It contains life-saving information, which can change the way you live. I'm sure you will find this book to be as informative as I did, and I am equally sure the suggestions and recommendations can help your prostate disorders as effectively as they did my friends.

Miraculous Breakthrough's practical approach to problems that so many face is most welcome. This book is a necessary addition to any home medical library."

Elena Groth, N.D.
Naturopathic physician:

"Exhaustively researched, very well-written, filled with life-saving information: a gold mine of advice and suggestions." These were my impressions of William Fischer's latest book, *Miraculous Breakthroughs*. He has succeeded in producing an intelligently written and highly sensitive volume on a topic not easily spoken of - the prostate and its effect on a man's emotional and physical health.

At long last, the public has a book it deserves on a subject too long neglected. *Miraculous Breakthroughs* explains why the tiny prostate gland looms so large in the health of men - especially men in their 40s and beyond.

This book is a keeper, to be read over and over again and used as a reference. It s advice is not only easy to implement, but inexpensive as well. It outlines modern medical techniques while showing low-cost alternative methods to achieving good health.

Ladies cannot afford to ignore this book, either - so packed is it with information vital to their own health and happiness."

C.H., a prostate patient:

"Several years ago I developed some problems with my prostate gland. The troubles looked innocent enough at first, but they eventually grew and the situation got more serious.

Someone loaned me a copy of *Miraculous Breakthroughs*. I had to admit, I was skeptical at first. I started off with some of your suggestions. Well, before I knew it, my problem had eased up. My doctor surely was surprised (shocked would be a better word) and I made sure I always checked with him every so often. Like I said, I was skeptical.

My prostate problems are gone, I'm happier than I've ever been and believe it or not, I feel I have the energy of someone half my age! Bless you!"

C.C.N., prostate patient:

"The doctor told me only surgery would help my problem. Naturally, I was reluctant to undergo a prostate operation.

I bought the book *Miraculous Breakthroughs* and learned there were sound natural alternatives to surgery. I immediately put your advice into use. My wife made fun of me at first, but she's not laughing now!

Just last week, my doctor told me the inflammation was so slight that the operation would not be needed. What a wonderful alternative to surgery! And, by the way, after following some of your advice on diet and exercise, I feel years younger. I think I may have found myself a new life."

F.Z., prostate patient:

"At 67, I developed a prostate problem. My friends told me it was a natural part of aging.

I picked up your book and was astonished to learn that even at my age I can avoid these problems. I bought some of those natural products you mentioned in the book and started eating better. My wife and I started walking every day.

You guessed it! I haven't had any more problems. For me, it really was a Miraculous Breakthrough.

I bought a copy for my son, who is in his early 40s. Maybe he can avoid prostate problems altogether."

Mrs. A.F.C., wife of a prostate patient:

"I can't thank you enough for your book *Miraculous Breakthroughs*. My husband had suffered from impotency for quite a while, but was too embarrassed to seek medical help. I bought your book and read it myself.

Imagine my surprise when I discovered that some prescription drugs can cause impotency! The medication my husband was taking appeared in your book. I showed this to him and he finally agreed to talk with his doctor. The doctor was only too happy to change his prescription.

Today, we are enjoying a truly loving marriage. Thank you so much.

By the way, my husband showed your book to the doctor, who thought it was very good, extremely well-researched, and of great benefit."

J.C.B., prostatitis patient:

"I'm not a health expert or any type of nutritional specialist. I am just an average guy - a guy who used to suffer from prostatitis.

But thanks to William Fischer's latest book, *Miraculous Breakthroughs*, I no longer am bothered by my prostate. I spent literally years searching for a doctor who could help me, but I found no relief. Finally, I gave up and resigned myself to living with the pain.

My wife bought me a copy of *Miraculous Breakthroughs*, but I was sure it would be of no use to me. Boy, was I wrong! There was so much sound advice, I can't imagine any man not finding something that agrees with his body and his lifestyle. I was thrilled to discover that two products worked especially well for me. The answer to my problem was so simple."

Chapter 1

What Is a Prostate Gland?

The male prostate gland weighs barely an ounce and is only the size of a walnut, but it has a great effect on the male reproductive system - and the self-images of thousands of men who feel its less-than-positive effects as their years add up.

The prostate gland is a doughnut-shaped organ that sits at the base of every man's bladder. It produces a component of male semen, the fluid responsible for carrying and keeping alive male sperm cells. If the prostate fails to function properly, a man may not only experience problems with sexual function, but will very likely have difficulty with urination. If left untreated, some prostate malfunctions can become life-threatening.

No man can afford to ignore his prostate. Indeed, awareness of this little organ has increased in recent years. Public figures like Senate Republican leader Bob Dole and Mississippi Governor Kirk Fordice went public with their diagnoses and recoveries from prostate illnesses - and rock star Frank Zappa and actors Telly Savalas and Bill Bixby died recently in their prime ages from prostate cancer.

The bulk of America's "Baby Boom" generation is reaching middle-age— the prime time for prostate trouble. Benign prostate hypertrophy, a non-fatal but bothersome enlargement of the gland, will affect half of all men over 40, and three-quarters of men over 65.

Even more frightening is the possibility of prostate cancer; a slow-growing cancer that will strike one man in 10. It will kill 35,000 American men this year, the American Cancer Institute says, even though diagnostic tests and treatments are widely available.

The number of reported prostate cases doubled between 1973 and 1990 - perhaps because of increased awareness and sophisticated diagnostics. And prostate cancer, for some unknown reason, is 25 percent more likely to strike African-American men than whites. Its incidence rises with age, so most men with prostate cancer die of old age rather than the disease.

All medical diagnoses and treatments should come from a licensed medical doctor. But men concerned about prostate health can lessen their suffering and hasten their recoveries by studying how diet, exercise and lifestyle changes can positively effect them. Men from other cultures have for centuries found prostate relief and even cures for cancerous growths through methods that American doctors may not have heard of. Some of these are outlined in this book.

But as always - common sense and professional guidance are recommended.

An Anatomy Lesson

When the prostate gland is healthy, it is a truly remarkable little organ. It doesn't only produce seminal fluid, it acts as a "storehouse" for male sperm.

The Prostate
What It Is and What It Does

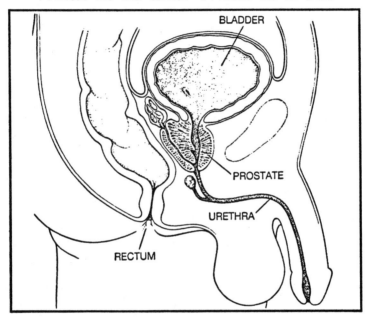

The prostate and the urinary tract share an outlet to the outside world, a tube known as the urethra - the reason that urine and semen come from the same opening at the end of the penis. Because this tube passes directly through the "doughnut hole" in the center of the prostate gland, enlargement of the gland can narrow the exit tube - thus causing the urinary problems familiar to so many men.

From "Prostate Problems," by Charles E. Shapiro, M.D., and Kathleen Doheny, Dell Surgical Library.

Sperm are too tiny to see without a microscope. They are dark, tadpole-shaped cells that carry a man's genetic information. They are custom designed to make the trip out of a man's body, into a woman's reproductive system and, if all goes according to biology, unite with a female ovum to create a new life.

Sperm cells are produced in a man's *testis* (see page 139), a small egg-shaped organ contained inside the scrotum, a bag of skin and sinew that hangs below the penis. After they are fully formed, sperm cells travel up the *vas deferens* to the prostate, where they are coated with a protective alkaline sheath. Without this chemical protection, sperm couldn't survive the acid environment of a woman's vagina.

The Hormones Do Their Part

At birth, the male prostate gland is only the size of a grain of barley. It doesn't begin growing until the onset of puberty, when *testosterone*, a sex-related chemical called a hormone, is produced in the nearby testes and signals the prostate to develop. The organ grows until about the age of 20, when the man reaches his full height.

Sexual arousal triggers a cellular exodus inside men with normal testosterone levels.

Sperm produced in the testes make a long journey upward, through yards of tiny tubes that lead to the prostate. Along the way they are supplied with high-energy milk sugar by the *seminal vesicles*, which then send the sperm for their alkaline coating of semen at the prostate gland. The finished product is sent through the ejaculatory duct, and from there into the *urethra*.

When orgasm occurs, the prostate initiates a rhythmic series of contractions, or squeezes, around the urethra - a process known as ejaculation. The muscle contraction propels three or four bursts of semen outward at intervals of about one second.

Frontal View of Prostate and Pubis

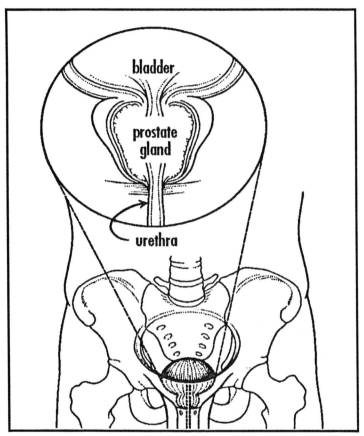

From "Prostate Problems," by Charles E. Shapiro, M.D., and Kathleen Doheny, Dell Surgical Library.

When arousal is triggered but orgasm is delayed, an uncomfortable condition called *prostatic congestion* - or "blue balls" - can occur. Doctors don't agree on the risks of physical damage from this condition. But they do say relief is always close to hand - release of the semen through masturbation is the usual cure.

How Age Changes the Prostate

It is not unusual for a man's prostate to become larger as he grows older. By age 65, three out of four men suffer with some kind of prostate disorder. The presence of androgens - male hormones - makes the prostate grow, and these are chemicals most men wouldn't want to do without.

Simple changes in body chemistry create the prostate enlargement. The changing body uses hormones, medications, food and other chemicals in new configurations, and organs sometimes receive "false messages" and react in ways that don't seem to make biological sense.

Upper Part of Urogenital System
(DETAIL)

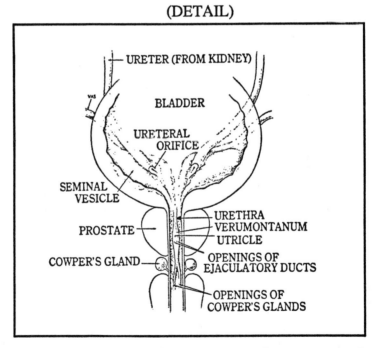

Statistics show that the average man's prostate begins growing at age 40, and begins to cause trouble of some kind by the time he reaches age 50. After that age, one in three men will require medical help for his prostate. In most cases, the symptoms are not pronounced until the condition is well-advanced.

Sometimes, the problem is easily solved. Urinary difficulty, one of the trademarks of prostate trouble, can also have other causes.

Men in their 60s and 70s sometimes find their urinary problems solved when they stop taking antihistamine medicine for colds or allergies. These drugs can cause contraction of the smooth muscle that surrounds the bladder neck and the prostate, which causes "urinary shutdown." Antihistamines don't seem to affect young men the same way. However, overindulgence in alcohol, especially beer, can cause acute urine retention in men of any age.

Prostatitis

The most simple-to-treat prostate problem is called *acute prostatitis*, or inflammation of the prostate. This bacterial condition affects old and young men alike, and is easily spotted by rapid onset of painful urination, pain at the base of the penis, presence of a cloudy fluid at the tip of the penis and a fever and chills.

Men with these symptoms should see a doctor immediately, as the symptoms can also indicate venereal disease. Treatment is a simple series of antibiotics.

Chronic Prostatitis is a similar form of prostate inflammation that is more difficult to treat. There is seldom a bacterial cause for the condition, which creates a need to urinate frequently, a lessened desire for sex and sometimes impotency - the inability to sustain an erection. Onset of chronic prostatitis is hard to pin down, because symptoms appear slowly and sometimes fade for months at a time.

The emotional toll of chronic prostatitis may be its most disturbing symptom. The sufferer may feel hopeless or depressed at his prospects for recovery, and his lack of sex drive may become a self-defeating resignation to permanent impotence.

Because of its sporadic nature, some doctors hesitate to treat chronic prostatitis with surgery or drugs. Many men find relief simply by talking about the problem with an understanding counselor, clergyman or companion. Others find that a good exercise program brings welcome relief. Others can get help through herbal cures and soothing baths, some of which are detailed later in this volume.

Chapter 2

Benign Prostatic Hypertrophy

Benign Prostatic Hypertrophy (BPH): Causes, Symptoms, Medical Treatments

Jim R., a 57-year-old personnel administrator, knows how many tiles there are along the baseboards in both his bathrooms. He'd counted them over and over while he waited to finish urinating.

He'd spent so much time in the john in the past few months he'd started to feel like a stranger in the rest of the house.

"I thought I'd broken a gasket there for a while," Jim said. "I'd have just laid back down after going to the bathroom for the second time in the night, and I'd feel like I had to go again. I couldn't make it through the second quarter of a ball game before I'd have to leave the room. It was getting embarrassing. And then it started to hurt."

Jim dislikes doctors and hospitals, but he swallowed his fear long enough to visit his family doctor.

After a physical that included a blood test and a digital rectal exam, Jim's doctor gave him the news.

"I just sat there and wondered, what the heck is benign prostatic hypertrophy?" Jim said.

Benign prostatic hypertrophy, or BPH, affects half of all men over 50, and three-quarters of those over 65. The condition is entirely unrelated to cancer, but in its extreme forms it can be life-threatening.

BPH is an enlargement of the prostate from double its normal size up to grapefruit proportions. Experts aren't sure what causes the condition. Some say a drop in testosterone levels. Others say it is caused by changes in how the body metabolizes hormones. Genetics, scarred-over injuries and surgeries - including vasectomy - have been linked to increased incidence of prostate enlargement. Some types of sexual activity can cause it to swell. Whatever its exact cause, the primary diagnosis is usually hormonal imbalance.

Comparison of Normal and Swollen Prostates

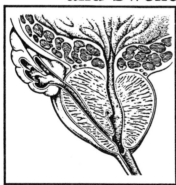 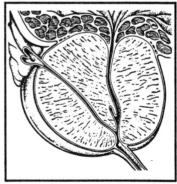

Normal Prostate   Enlarged Prostate

From "Prostate Problems," by Charles E. Shapiro, M.D., and Kathleen Doheny, Dell Surgical Library.

Prostatic hypertrophy is practically undetectable until its later stages, because it develops slowly over many years. As the enlargement progresses, though, the man may experience pain in the groin or lower back, or he may feel a slight discomfort when he sits down.

As the condition progresses, sexual performance may be effected. Ejaculation can become painful, and a man may find himself ejaculating prematurely. He may even have intermittent bouts of impotence.

Some patients find that their headache remedy, ulcer or bowel medicine or other commonly-used medications for depression or high blood-pressure are making their prostate disorders worse. A list of drugs that commonly complicate prostate problems appears in the appendix.

Other mens' prostates grow to a certain point and then stop. Enlargement doesn't necessarily mean the problem will become progressively worse. About 80 percent of men found to have mild BPH decide to delay treatment. Doctors call this option "watchful waiting," going about your ordinary routine while keeping a careful watch for changes. Some men see their symptoms improve spontaneously.

But not everyone is so lucky. For a man with a growing prostate, urination frequently becomes painful. Less urine is able to pass through the penis as the prostate slowly squeezes shut the urethra - the passageway between the bladder and penis. The prostate grows upward against the bladder, narrowing the duct which routes urine to the urethra. Sometimes urination slows to a trickle. The bladder feels uncomfortably full. The man finds himself waking up frequently in the night to drain off whatever he can.

This situation can become life-threatening if it is allowed to continue unchecked and "strangle" the urinary tract.

In a worst-case scenario, the urine sits in a distended bladder, the chances of infection increasing as time passes. The bladder becomes inflamed, bladder stones may form, and the urine backs up into the kidneys. This leads to complete kidney shutdown, which can create fatal uremic poisoning of the bloodstream.

Fortunately, medical intervention is almost certain before these dire straits are reached. The vast majority of men die WITH a prostate problem, not FROM one. The key to preventing the pain of BPH is early detection and treatment.

Some Prostate Warning Signs:
- Pain in prostate area
- Pain in the lower back
- Discomfort when sitting
- Painful urination
- Weak stream of urine
- Continual feeling of fullness in bladder
- Waking several times at night to urinate, with only a small amount voided
- Painful ejaculation
- Intermittent impotency
- Dribbling

Medical Diagnosis of BPH

Jim's initial doctor visit was just what he'd expected—a little unnerving. The questions were intense: How often do you urinate, day and night? How steady is the flow? Do you have to stand and wait a while before the flow starts?

How often do you have sexual intercourse? Do you have pain on ejaculation? But based on his answers, Jim's doctor ordered a full BPH evaluation.

His were only some of the methods doctors use to diagnose prostate troubles. Tests include the following:

Digital Rectal Examination

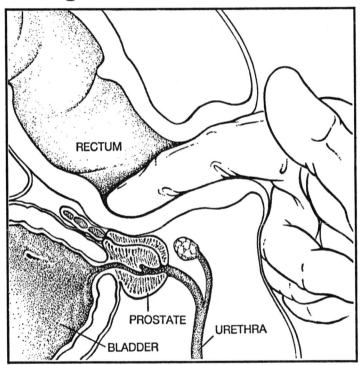

The doctor feels inside the rectum with a gloved finger. Because part of the prostate lies against the wall of the colon, doctors can detect abnormalities and tender spots with the touch of a finger.

Cystoscopy: A special viewing tube is inserted through the penis, which enables the doctor to view the obstruction and evaluate any damage the obstruction may have done inside the bladder. (A local anesthetic is used.)

Postvoidal and urine flow measures: Sometimes doctors have a patient drink a large amount of fluid, to create a full bladder. The man then urinates into a funnel with a flow meter attached. This records the speed of the urine stream and the amount of urine produced. This test can determine if there is an obstruction in the urethra, and can also provide an important "baseline" measure for later tests.

A postvoidal residual measure determines the amount of urine that remains in the bladder after urination. This is done by inserting a catheter into the bladder, or by ultrasound, an imaging technique that bounces high-frequency sound waves off the liquid inside the bladder.

Ultrasound scans, or Intravenous Pyelography (IVP): are not usually performed right away. This technique evaluates the kidneys and other urinary organs to determine where the trouble is. IVPs require fasting and injection of a radioactive dye into a vein. A doctor then shoots X-rays as the dye makes its way through the urinary tract.

Ultrasound images are configured on computer screens, giving the doctor a clear view of internal organs without use of invasive procedures. These tests rule out prostate ailments like tumors, prostatitis and urinary tract infections.

Prostate-Specific Antigen (PSA) Blood Test: A laboratory test that determines the level of a prostatic protein in the blood stream. Doctors routinely use this test to make sure the swollen prostate isn't cancerous.

Medical Treatments for BPH

Millions of dollars and hours have been poured into research on BPH - its causes and cures. Research has found three major options for men whose symptoms are intolerable and whose medical work-ups indicate a BPH-related blockage of the urinary tract.

These are medications, surgery or "investigational methods," treatments that are still under study but are currently performed by qualified doctors.

Medications are usually the first step in dealing with a surly prostate.

Alpha Blockers: Hawk-eyed doctors in Wisconsin in 1991 found a link between blood-pressure medication and relief from BPH symptoms. Terazosin (brand name "Hytrin") is usually prescribed for high blood pressure. It works by dilating, or widening, the blood vessels. A 1991 study at the Medical College of Wisconsin found the drug also relaxed the muscles at the neck of the bladder, bringing relief of blocked urine flow to 59 percent of BPH-affected men on a large (10 mg) dosage. Prazosin (Minipress), and doxasozin (Cardura) had similar effects on BPH patients.

The downside of alpha-blockers is their many side effects, which include sharp drops in blood pressure, dizziness, tiredness and impotence. Not everyone can take these drugs.

Another class of medications now growing in popularity is called the *Luteinizing Hormone-Releasing Hormone (LH-RH) agonists*. They include *leuprolide* (Lupron) and *nafarelin acetate* (Synarel). They work by blocking production of testosterone, the male hormone that signals the prostate to grow. They are usually used to treat prostate cancer. The medicine is injected once a month, and works to shrinking the prostate gland by cutting off testosterone.

LH-RH agonists almost always produce impotence. Other side effects include headaches and hot flashes.

Flutamide (Eulexin) also shrinks the prostate through

hormone manipulation. But its side effects include stomach upset and breast development.

One promising - and heavily advertised - new drug is *Finesteride* (Proscar), a prostate shrinker discovered through a group of Caribbean natives a researcher found in the Dominican Republic.

In the mid 1970s, the scientist told his colleagues about the ethnic group, none of whom ever developed BPH or male-pattern baldness. Closer examination of the group found a genetic trait that created a deficiency of a blood protein called 5-alpha reductase. This protein usually interacts with testosterone to signal prostate growth. Without it, the natives' prostates remained small throughout adulthood.

Over several years, chemists at Merck Pharmaceuticals Co. developed *Finesteride*, (marketed as Proscar), a chemical that blocks production of 5-alpha reductase. Clinical trials have shown about a third of the men who take the drug experience improved urine flow and marked prostatic shrinkage.

Disadvantages include a long waiting period before results are seen, occasional impotence and an indefinite effectiveness - one study found that four months after discontinuing the drug, prostate symptoms had returned to their pre-treatment conditions. It simply doesn't work for two-thirds of the men who try it.

Another drawback to *Finesteride* is its effect on blood chemistry. Researchers say it lowers levels of other prostate proteins that are important to cancer diagnoses.

Finesteride can also effect women. Women of childbearing age, pregnant women and those who may someday bear children are warned against handling the tablets, as the chemical can pass into the system through skin contact and cause abnormal sexual development in male fetuses.

Men who use *Finesteride* are warned to use condoms if they have intercourse with a fertile partner, as their semen can have a similar effect: Male children conceived by *Finesteride* patients may be born with malformed sex organs.

Doctors are also experimenting with combinations of finesteride and alpha-blockers. Studies are now being performed that compare the double-up approach to use of *Finesteride* alone.

But sometimes medicine doesn't do the job, or the symptoms are too advanced for pharmaceutical treatment. At this point, most medical doctors recommend prostate surgery.

Surgery

Dr. Charles Shapiro and Kathleen Doheny give detailed descriptions of surgical prostate treatments in their 1993 book "The Well Informed Patient's Guide to Prostate Problems." Available options are simply outlined here.

Standard prostate surgeries include *Open Prostatectomy, Transurethral Resection (TURP); Transurethral Incision, (TUIP); balloon dilation;* and *laser surgery.*

Open prostatectomy is the most radical surgical procedure, and is usually reserved for very large prostates or cancerous glands. Usually using general anesthesia, a doctor removes the offending tissue through an incision in the man's lower abdomen. Prostatectomy patients can expect a hospital stay of up to a week. About 85 percent of prostatectomy patients are left impotent; 27 percent are partially incontinent.

Transurethral Resection, or TURP, is called "the gold standard" in prostate surgeries in several medical texts.

Transurethral Resection (TURP) Removes Overgrown Prostate Tissue

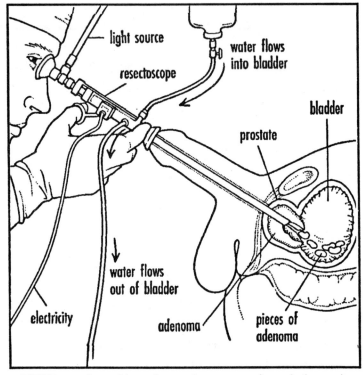

TURP consists of inserting an instrument through the penis and cutting away the overgrown prostate tissue. There is no skin incision. The operation takes 30 minutes to two hours, and usually requires general or spinal anesthetic. Samples of the excised tissue are then analyzed for cancer growth.

From "Prostate Problems," by Charles E. Shapiro, M.D.,
and Kathleen Doheny, Dell Surgical Library.

A curious side effect of TURP is "retrograde ejaculation." Because the incision traumatizes the tubes that carry semen to the urethra, most mens' bodies instead will, after surgery, send the semen backward into the bladder instead of out the usual exit. The ejaculate is then harmlessly eliminated with the urine. Sexual sensation is not effected by the surgery or retrograde ejaculation, doctors say, even though some couples find these "dry orgasms" a little disconcerting.

TUIP, or *transurethral incision*, uses the same instrument and anesthesia as a TURP. It is usually used on smaller prostates and younger men, and involves no incision or removal of tissue. Patients report less retrograde ejaculation with this operation - only about one in four are effected.

A very few doctors now use lasers, balloons and ultra-sound techniques to perform similar operations. Lasers are intense light beams that can burn away tissue without causing bleeding. Doctors report less bleeding and a quicker post-operative recovery time, but these high-tech, investigational procedures are still too expensive for many patients, and their long-term effectiveness isn't yet determined.

Laser Surgery of the Enlarged Prostate

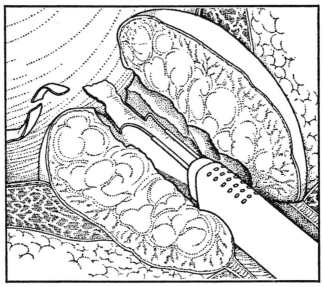

From "Prostate Problems," by Charles E. Shapiro, M.D.,
and Kathleen Doheny, Dell Surgical Library.

There are medical drawbacks to these less-invasive and quicker surgeries. Because no tissue is removed from the prostate, doctors can't test for cancer cells. And the long-term benefits of transurethral incisions are questioned, since many patients must return for more surgery when their prostates again enlarge and block urinary flow.

Balloon dilation of the prostate is another popular treatment, and is especially useful for prostate sufferers whose other health problems make surgery risky. Using an instrument similar to the TURP, a doctor inserts the tip of a carefully measured balloon into the prostate through the urethra. As the balloon inflates, it spreads open the prostate, widening the passage to the bladder by splitting the interfering prostate tissue.

Balloon Dilation of the Prostate - *Deflated*

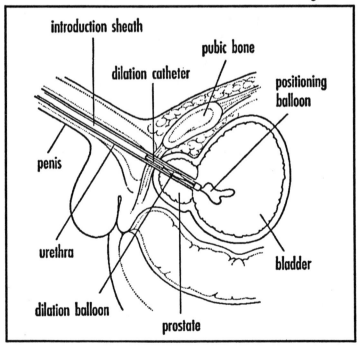

Balloon Dilation of the Prostate - *Inflated*

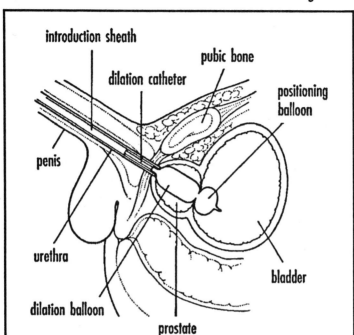

introduction sheath

pubic bone

dilation catheter

positioning balloon

penis

urethra

dilation balloon

prostate

bladder

From "Prostate Problems," by Charles E. Shapiro, M.D., and Kathleen Doheny, Dell Surgical Library.

Studies show that balloon dilation brings long-term relief to up to 60 percent of patients, but many must return for retreatment. Also, no prostate tissue is removed for routine cancer analysis. The procedure is sometimes done on an outpatient basis.

As with any surgical procedure, there are certain risks of bleeding, anesthesia reactions, infection, scarring or postoperative incontinence. Ten to 15 percent of men report problems with sexual impotence or loss of desire. As a rule, the older the patient, the more likely he is to experience sexual problems after prostate surgery. Impotence treatments will be covered in a later chapter.

Other medical techniques are still under study, and probably won't be generally available until the mid-1990s, Shapiro says.

These include *stents*, slender tubes made of surgical titanium, gold-coated steel or "super alloys," which are easily implanted in the urethra. Major work on stent procedures is now underway at the Mayo Clinic and Columbia Presbyterian Medical Center in New York.

The Intra-Prostatic Stent

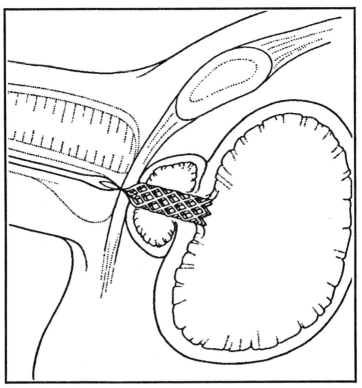

The stent pushes back the prostate, opens the urethra and relieves urinary problems.

From "Prostate Problems," by Charles E. Shapiro, M.D., and Kathleen Doheny, Dell Surgical Library.

Hyperthermia or Microwave treatments use heat to shrink prostate tissue. One procedure, called a *Prostatron*, uses an ultrasound-guided catheter to deliver a blast of 110-degree heat to the prostate. The urethra is protected from the heat by water, which is kept steadily flowing around and through the catheter. Doctors say the treated tissue shrinks during the weeks following the procedure, bringing slow-but-steady relief of urinary difficulty.

Other microwave studies have involved repeated treatments or use of a rectally-administered device, but tissue damage and ineffective delivery of the microwaves made the therapies unusable, according to a review in the *Journal of Andrology*.

Doctors and researchers don't rely solely on chemicals and surgeries for treatment. They constantly search for new solutions to this age-old problem.

Because medicine is rapidly developing, the procedures outlined here may have been developed while the book went to press. Those interested in the latest studies on BPH treatments may contact the urology department of their community teaching hospital or university medical center.

Chapter 3

Nature's Way of Dealing with Enlarged Prostates

We Americans are fascinated by medical science and high technology. We hold our doctors in awe, and take their word as Gospel truth - sometimes to our own detriment. We look to them for quick solutions to health problems we develop through years of bodily neglect or abuse.

Most thinking people know there are other solutions to medical problems - sources of relief that lie far from the antiseptic atmosphere of the pharmacy or operating theater. Relief, and sometimes a cure, can be found in nature. This statement that can be safely made without casting doubt on the expertise of the doctors who study prostate and urinary tract functions.

Many healthy men say their lack of prostate problems is due to good common sense - eating right, exercising, taking in the right balance of vitamin and minerals. But to the man accustomed to high-fat meals and a low-energy lifestyle, surgery may seem an easier alternative than a lifestyle change... until his doctor schedules a prostate procedure for him!

We all know that a good diet can provide your body with the vitality needed for a healthy, active life. Perhaps the role of diet is best illustrated by that raspy-voiced, muscle-bound cartoon sailor man, Popeye.

Popeye's superhuman feats and hair's breadth rescues were fueled by spinach — the lowly leafy-green he forever carried, canned, in his bosom or back pocket. After tearing open the tin and swallowing down its contents, Popeye's strength bounded forth in a frenzy of bulging biceps and karate kicks.

Popeye illustrates that old saw: "You are what you eat." Diet can, indeed, provide us with seemingly unlimited strength and energy. The only thing wrong with Popeye's spinach was the can. He really should have been eating it fresh.

But what does a good diet have to do with the prostate gland?

Health comes from the inside out. No one can appear outwardly healthy if he isn't putting healthy things inside. A proper diet provides the right nutrients for every organ of the body - including the prostate.

Processed and refined foods contain chemical flavor enhancers and preservatives that are carefully controlled by the Food and Drug Administration - because in large doses or under certain storage conditions, these chemicals are poisonous to humans. It's no surprise that study after study finds that cutting out processed foods and increasing intake

of natural and fresh food brings about better health —
including a healthier prostate.

Researchers are studying several natural substances that
are known to shrink the prostate - and even cure cases of
benign prostatic hypertrophy.

Zinc

For more than 50 years science has known that seminal
fluid from a healthy prostate contains a high concentration
of zinc. One ejaculation may contain nearly all the zinc
absorbed by the body in one day.

Zinc deficiency in males can have serious consequences.
It can lead to infertility and, in severe cases, impotency.
Some evidence also shows that a lack of zinc may be the
culprit in cases of chronic prostatitis.

In a study at Chicago's Cook County Hospital, the zinc
content of semen samples from chronic prostatitis patients
was measured against samples taken from normal, healthy
men. The prostatitis sufferers' semen contained 50 mgs of
zinc per milliliter. The normal samples contained an average
of 448 mgs per milliliter - more than nine times that of the
prostatitis sufferers.

In another study, 200 male patients with prostatitis were
given zinc supplements. With doses of 11 to 34 mg. a day
over four months, more than 70 percent of the men reported
their symptoms disappeared.

In St. Louis, a Washington University School of Medicine study indicated that zinc has antibacterial properties that
may protect the prostate from infections. However, men
already infected with bacterial prostatitis did not respond to
zinc therapy.

The US Recommended Daily Allowance of zinc is 15mg a day for adults. Although some nutritionists disagree, many doctors say it is difficult to get enough zinc from a normal diet. Shellfish are the best dietary source of zinc. Oysters contain between 70 and 100 grams of zinc apiece — and their reputation as an aphrodisiac is legendary!

As a daily supplement, men should take no more than 30 mg of zinc each day. Not all zinc taken into the body is absorbed, and too much may interfere with the body's processing of other minerals like iron and copper.

Other sources of zinc include eggs, cheese, legumes, seeds, nuts, peas, corn, carrots, brown rice, garlic, onions, wheat germ, whole grains and brewer's yeast; however, eggs and cheese should be eaten in moderation. Their fat and cholesterol contents have been linked to heart disease.

Selenium

Some researchers say selenium — another trace element the body needs in tiny amounts — is a good preventive medicine for prostate sufferers. It improves the blood's ability to deliver oxygen, keeps tissues elastic and firm, and also helps keep the eye retina healthy.

Cholesterol and the Prostate

High blood cholesterol levels have been linked to enlarged prostates in laboratory dogs by researchers at Rutgers University and New York's Metropolitan Hospital. (Man's Best Friend shares Man's characteristic prostate enlargement as he grows older - making him a good specimen for experimental prostate cures.)

Although tests are still preliminary, a Rutgers study showed that reducing cholesterol levels in older dogs resulted in a shrinkage of their enlarged prostates. The chief urologist at the New York hospital studied prostates from 100 men of all ages. She found that prostates with BPH symptoms had cholesterol counts an average of 80 percent higher than normal glands.

Mark Bricklin reports in his "Practical Encyclopedia of Natural Healing" on a recent American Health Foundation study of rural men in South Africa. These men typically eat only low-fat, whole foods, and have few prostate problems.

Dr. Peter Hill placed a group of South African volunteers on a typical American diet, complete with plenty of fats and meat. At the same time, a group of North American volunteers were put on a low-fat diet.

After three weeks, Dr. Hill found the Africans on the Western diet had a markedly higher number of hormones in their blood, while the North Americans on the low-fat diet showed a concurrent decrease in excreted hormones. In only three weeks, the high-risk American group had lowered its metabolic profile to match the original low-risk group.

"By changing diet, you can change hormonal metabolism," Hill told Bricklin. "And prostatic cancer seems to be a hormonally associated disease."

Essential Fatty Acids

Dr. W. Devrient, a German nutritionist whose work is well-known in Europe, believes that essential fatty acids are vital in healing and maintaining prostate tissue.

Research shows that men need five times the fatty acids women do, to help maintain the elasticity of cell tissue. Seeds, nuts and the oil from flaxseeds are all excellent sources of these important nutrients.

Devrient tells prostate patients to consume lots of seeds and nuts daily - especially pumpkin, squash and sesame seeds. Almonds, too, are a good source of fatty acids.

Pumpkin seeds and pumpkin seed oil are Devrient's favorites. He calls them "an inexhaustible source of vigor offered by Mother Nature."

Rick R., one of Devrient's patients, testifies to the effectiveness of this humble healer. He developed prostate problems when only 40 years old. His doctor recommended surgery, but Rick's brother had undergone a similar operation two years before. He'd advised Rick to avoid the procedure at any cost.

Instead, Rick began pumpkin seed therapy. He ate pumpkin seeds by the handful - about 20 or 30 pounds of seeds a year. It's been five years since the doctor ordered surgery, and Rick says he walks away from each checkup with a clean bill of health.

Flaxseed oil is an alternative for those who don't care for crunchy seeds and nuts, which are sometimes difficult for denture-wearers to chew. *Unrefined, cold-pressed flaxseed oil*, only one tablespoon per day mixed with unsweetened yogurt or low fat cottage cheese, is used throughout Europe in treatment of BPH. It is also used to treat *cancer, arteriosclerosis, arthritis* and *eczema.*

As shown in the chart that follows, the body converts the *linoleic* and *linolenic acids* in the *unrefined flaxseed oil* into prostaglandins, chemicals that are present in healthy prostates, seminal fluids, lungs, kidneys, thymus glands and brain tissues. Several prostaglandins act as vasodilators - opening up veins and capillaries and increasing blood flow.

Presence of Polyunsaturated Fatty Acids in Various Oils and Their Influence on Human Diseases

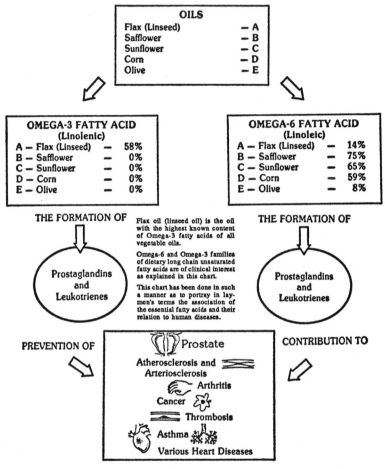

Flax oil (linseed oil) is the best seed oil for people with fatty degeneration, because the oil contains the largest amount of the most strongly dispersing essential fatty acid, the three times unsaturated linolenic acid (LNA = linolenic acid = Omega-3).

LNA helps to disperse from our tissues deposits of the saturated fatty acids and cholesterol, which like to aggregate and which make platelets sticky. (Platelets play an important role in blood coagulation and blood thrombus formation.) The oil has to be fresh, and not exposed to light, oxygen, and heat, because these three agent destroy the essential fatty acids very rapidly. Flax oil (linseed oil) should be *unrefined*, fresh, not older than 3 months after pressing.*

*From the complete "Guide to Fats and Oils in Health and Nutrition."

Los Angeles physician Dr. W.L. Cooper reported on an experimental *unrefined flaxseed oil* treatment administered to 19 prostate patients. Results included the following improvements:

- Increased sexual drive
- Increased energy
- Reduction in size of prostate gland
- Increased urination
- Less residual urine

Essential Fatty Acids Content of Common Vegetable Oils

Source	Fat Content Total %	Essential Fatty Acids Linolenic	Linoleic	Both Essentials Total %
Linseed[†]	35	58	14	72
Soybean	18	9	50	59
Pumpkin	47	15	42	57
Walnut	60	5	51	56
Rapeseed*	30	7	30	37
Safflower	59	0	75	
Sunflower	47	0	65	
Grape	Trace	0	71	
Corn	4	0	59	
Wheat Germ	10	0	54	
Sesame	49	0	54	
Rice Bran	10	0	35	
Cotton**	Trace	0	50	
Peanut***	47	0	29	

Continued

Essential Fatty Acids Content of
Common Vegetable Oils *Continued*

Source	Fat Content Total %	Essential Fatty Acids Linolenic	Linoleic	Both Essentials Total %
Almond	54	0	17	
Macadamia	71	0	10	
Cashew	41	0	6	
Olive	20	0	8	
Coconut	35	0	3	
Palm Kernel	35	0	3	

† Linseed (flaxseed) unrefined, cold-pressed
*Rapeseed (canola) contains toxic *erucic acid*
**Cottonseed contains common toxins
***Peanuts (damp) harbor a toxic fungus
Hemp (not listed because it is illegal in the U.S.) provides both essential fatty acids.

Bee Pollen

Many men who successfully treated their prostate symptoms with iron also swear by a supplement that seems to work well with zinc. *Bee pollen* - a natural substance created by honey bees to nourish their young, contains every nutrient known by doctors to maintain good health. Its positive effect on prostatitis is remarkable.

Nutritionists say bee pollen contains more than 5,000 enzymes and co-enzymes - far more than any other food. Enzymes are essential to healing and digestion, and are said to protect against premature aging. It is also packed with important vitamins, proteins and nucleic acids - some authorities call it "nature's perfect food."

HIGH DESERT ® HONEYBEE POLLENS™
CHEMICAL ANALYSIS

PROTEIN
7.1 GRAMS PER OZ (RDA 12 GRAMS)

Standard chemical analysis identifies only 18 of the 22 amino acids present in pollen.

AMINO ACIDS	MGs PER OZ
Cystine	36.855
Lysine	366.360
Histidine	138.590
Arginine	292.520
Aspartic	542.440
Threonine	236.856
Serine	289.680
Glutamic	585.040
Proline	505.520
Glycine	267.520
Alanine	309.560
Valine	280.592
Methionine	94.004
Isoleucine	230.040
Leucine	377.720
Tyrosine	139.440
Phenylalanine	236.850
Tryptophan	49.700

Note: "Realities of Nutrition" states a person using the RDA to choose protein foods might not get enough of all essential amino acids. Bee pollen contains all essential amino acids.

MINERALS	MGs PER OZ
Calcium	42.383
Iron	2.118
Potassium	158.675
Phosphorus	121.706
Sodium	2.693
Iodine (in MCGs)	6.237
Magnesium	27.675
Zinc	1.460
Copper	.221
Boron	.604
Barium	.136
Chromium (less than)	.010
Manganese	1.395
Strontium	.094

MISCELLANEOUS	GRAM PER OZ
Carbohydrates	5.15
Fiber	1.02
Reducing Sugars	8.25
Ash	.65
CALORIES PER OUNCE	.90

VITAMINS	MGs PER OZ
A - 232,470 I.U.*	
Alpha Carotene	.031
Beta Carotene	.122
B1 (Thiamine)	.198
B2 (Riboflavin)	.459
B3 (Niacin)	2.551
B^ (Pyridoxine)	.119
B12 (Cyanocobalamin)	.00002
Biotin	.002
Folic Acid	.201
Pantothenic Acid	.198
C - (Ascorbic Acid)	1.304
D - 9 I.U.*	
E - 2.194 I.U.*	
* International Units	

RUTIN - Abundant. (Not measured in analysis) Of great importance for capillary strength.

ENZYMES - Active enzymes are needed to digest and assimilate nutrients. Chemical analysis measures only three of the many present in bee pollen.

ENZYME	UNITS PER GRAM
Amylase (USP Units)	2.550
(Needed to break down starch)	
Protease (USP Units)	64.400
Needed to split proteins)	
Lipase (mm Units)	.085
(Needed to emulsify fats)	

FATTY ACIDS 2.807 GRAM/OZ

Essential fatty acids, with carbohydrates and sugars, supply our energy requirements.

- CHOLESTEROL - 0 PERCENT -

Bee pollen contains a higher content (11) of the healthful unsaturated fatty acids as opposed to saturated (9).

NOTE: Bee pollen also contains elements science is not yet able to isolate and identify. Some authorities believe it is precisely these elements often called the "magic" of the bee, which make bee pollen so effective.

NOTE: This important chemical analysis was conducted by an independent testing laboratory on the justly famous enzyme-active *High-Desert® PollenS™* blend. It does not apply to any other brand of bee pollen in the world. If you see this analysis, or any portion thereof, reprinted elsewhere you may be certain proprietary material is being used both incorrectly and illegally to persuade you another product has the same documented high nutrient count as blended High-Desert®. Source: C.C. Pollen Company, Arizona

Dr. Bernard C. Jensen, one of America's foremost natural nutritionists, said in his book *Nature Has A Remedy* that "much has been said about pollen helping glands in the body. All experiments on animals show it prolongs life - and helps to keep the glands in good order."

Researchers at the Nagasaki University School of Medicine in Japan and the University of Lund in Sweden did independent studies of *bee pollen* and prostate problems. Both reported marked reduction in prostatic swelling and inflammation, even in severe cases of *prostatitis*. Neither study reported any adverse side effects.

Of the 172 prostate-diseased men in a Swedish-German study in 1988, all who were treated with oral doses of *bee pollen* reported a cessation of symptoms.

Bee pollen therapy began about 40 years ago in Sweden, where beekeepers discovered how much better they felt after indulging in the natural tonic.

Dr. Erik Ask-Upmark M.D., a professor at the University of Upsala, learned of the substance from a beekeeping patient in 1957. The patient had intermittent bouts of *prostatitis,* accompanied by severe localized symptoms and high fevers. He'd found no relief from doctors — and Dr. Ask-Upmark could offer no solutions.

The patient decided to take *bee pollen* as a general tonic, to build up his strength for a scheduled prostate surgery. Very shortly after beginning the *bee pollen* doses, the man noticed that his *prostatitis* was gone.

He continued taking the pollen, and his symptoms only returned once - after he'd stopped taking the pollen for two weeks. His urologist canceled the surgery.

Ludwik Frangor was 70 when he discovered the benefits of *bee pollen*. At that time, his heart was so diseased his doctor wouldn't let him mow the lawn. He had given up on sex - he was widowed, so his impotence no longer bothered him. As his condition deteriorated, his son suggested he move to a nursing home for 24-hour-care. The suggestion changed his life — Ludwik decided he wasn't ready to die yet.

"From then on, I made *honeybee pollen* the one unvarying and essential foundation of my rejuvenation program," he said. "This perfect live food has restored my manhood, brought me back to full vigor... I am never sick."

Frangor celebrated his 94th birthday in 1989 with a cross-country ski trip.

Studies at Yugoslavia's University of Sarajevo showed that bee pollen therapy aids in cases of prostatitis and impotency - and may also cure some cases of male infertility. *Bee pollen* administered to a group of infertile men produced a measurable increase in sperm production. Scientists credited a gonadotropin hormone in the pollen with the gland stimulation.

Dr. James Van Fleet routinely treats BPH and *prostatitis* patients with *bee pollen*. He told of a patient named Bill G., whose *prostate gland* was so swollen he visited the restroom every 20 minutes. The problem was costing him much sleep and work productivity, the pain in his lower abdomen and back was becoming unbearable.

Dr. Van Fleet gave Bill *bee pollen*. He recommended a dose of eight capsules a day, two with each meal and two at bedtime. In less than a month, Bill's most severe symptoms had eased, and within two months he was sleeping through the night again.

Scientists in this country have tried without success to scientifically duplicate *bee pollen*. Its unique combination of vitamins, minerals, amino acids, hormones, carbohydrates and fatty acids - all in just the right proportions - has left chemists flummoxed.

Natural nutritionists say that many kinds of *bee pollen* are available at natural foods markets, but savvy customers should look for granules or capsules made from *"high desert"* sources. This type of pollen is made from many different types of plants indigenous to unspoiled areas of Montana and the Dakotas of the western United States. It is not damaged through heat-processing, and is free of industrial pollution.

Larry R., 65, visited Dr. Van Fleet when his family doctor told him his prostate gland should be surgically removed. Van Fleet's tests revealed Larry had a zinc deficiency. The doctor prescribed his usual eight capsules of *bee pollen*, but also had Larry take 10 mg. of zinc with each meal.

Within 10 days, Larry noticed improvement. After a month, all signs of prostate problems had disappeared.

Dr. Norman Meyers ran into a stubborn problem with patient Ed J., 79. Although he took the same dosages of zinc and *bee pollen* as Larry R., his condition did not improve.

Essential fatty acids, in the form of *unrefined, coldpressed flaxseed oil*, proved to be the missing element in Ed's diet. When he consumed a tablespoon of the oil in yogurt or low fat cottage cheese each day, his symptoms responded immediately.

Drs. Van Fleet and Meyers say that even men whose prostates are healthy should follow their nutritional recommendations as a preventative measure. The table at the end of this chapter shows the amounts of supplements to take, and when to take them. All are available from any reputable natural foods store.

Prostatitis Cures: Helpful Herbs

John Heinermann, an anthropologist and herbalist from Utah, has several suggestions for men who suffer with prostatitis, the bacterial or the chronic.

Heinermann says *Goldenseal root* is especially helpful in reducing *prostatitis* symptoms. A recipe for Goldenseal tea is included later in this volume - he recommends three half-cups every 4 hours. *Fluid goldenseal extract* is also available at natural foods stores, dosage is 15 drops three times a day. Those who prefer capsules should take two every five hours.

Chaparral is another herb that helps a swollen prostate. Heinermann recommends one cup of *chaparral tea* twice daily; 10 drops of fluid extract three times a day; or 4 capsules each day.

Yarrow and *mallow* are two anti-inflammatory herbs that some prostate sufferers swear by - they soothe pain and burning sensations. Users should drink two cups of tea per day or swallow 4 capsules of either herb daily.

Heinermann stresses the importance of easy exercise and a diet high in fatty acids, zinc, fruits and vegetables. He also recommends use of "liquid chlorophyll," a green make-it-yourself concoction that is packed with vitamins and minerals needed for a healthy body and prostate.

To make the mixture, simply puree Romaine lettuce leaves, parsley and celery in a blender, juicer or food processor. Strain and drink a half-glass at a time. The juice is also available in pre-made form at health food stores under the name "Kyo-Green."

Prescription for a
Healthy Prostate

Supplement	Breakfast	Lunch	Dinner	Bed
Bee pollen capsules*	2	2	2	2
Zinc tablets	10 mg	10 mg	10 mg	—
Flaxseed Oil**	One tablespoon at breakfast, mixed with lowfat cottage cheese, unsweetened yogurt or tofu.			

* Or 1 to 3 tablespoons granulated bee pollen per day.
** *Only Unrefined, cold-pressed flaxseed oil is recommended.*

Chapter 4

Flower Pollen and Royal Jelly
New Angles on Old Cures

Nature offers an abundance of relief to ailments of almost every part of the human body. Indeed, pharmacologists frequently find new medicines by examining folk remedies. *Digitalis*, a well-known treatment for heart rhythm dysfunctions, comes from the common *Foxglove*, a wild flower Native Americans used for healing for centuries. Bread mold, used by Dutch and German immigrants to bring down fevers and heal infected cuts, was later used to form *penicillin* - the first antibiotic "miracle drug."

Many Europeans swear by another such discovery made "in the back yard." *Flower pollen extract*, a potent and proven help in cases of *prostate enlargement*, comes from eight species of wildflowers that grow in the Scania district of southern Sweden. This is not the same as the *bee pollen* discussed in chapter 3: *flower pollen* isn't taken in and digested by bees before being processed.

Cernitin, or *Cernitex,* the major ingredient in flower pollen, increases body tissues' resistance to invasion by outside agents, thus creating an anti-inflammatory effect. The other pollens work to promote urination, which is typically suppressed by prostate disorders.

Although the word "pollen" might make one think of watering eyes and itchy noses, all allergens are processed out of the *flower pollen* before they are administered to patients. Double-blind tests performed by urologists at Upsala University in Sweden examined the effects of a substance on a group of BPH patients as compared against a similar group taking a harmless "placebo," or sugar pill. They found the *flower pollen* extract to be authentically beneficial to 90 percent of the men who took it.

Long-term use of the substance has shown no ill effects. Even those whose prostates did not shrink under treatment reported drops in the intensity of their symptoms. 76 percent of those tested reported relief from dysuria, or difficult and painful urination. 89 percent said their urine streams had increased markedly with the *flower pollen* therapy.

These improvements are due to the extract's contracting effect on the smooth "detrusor" muscle, which is responsible for emptying the bladder.

Flower pollen also suppresses production of androgenic hormones in the prostate - the same hormones suppressed by *alpha-blocker* medications discussed in chapter 2. The *alpha-blockers,* however, suppress the hormones produced in the testes, and their use sometimes results in impotence and breast development. Because the *flower pollen* works specifically on the prostate, no such side effects have been reported by its users.

Questions and Answers About Flower Pollen Extract Tablets and Their Therapeutic Effectiveness For Diseases of The Prostate Gland

Q. 1 What is Flower Pollen Extract?

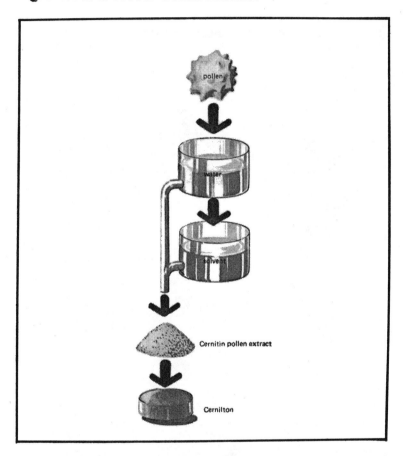

A Flower Pollen Extract is a therapeutic agent for diseases of the prostate whose main ingredient is Cernitin (or Cernitex) pollen extract, extracted from the pollen of 8 plant species grown in the Scania district of South Sweden.

This substance has traditionally been used in Sweden for reinforcing physical strength as an anti-influenza agent, nutrient, tonic etc. Its effectiveness on prostatitis was discovered by Ask-Upmark (Upsala University) in 1960 and was later confirmed in a double blind test. Since its discovery excellent results have been achieved in improving symptoms of chronic prostatitis and prostatic hypertrophy. Furthermore, since allergens are removed, it does not cause allergies and is a drug with extremely few side effects.

Q. 2 Why should Flower Pollen Extract be effective on diseases of the prostate?

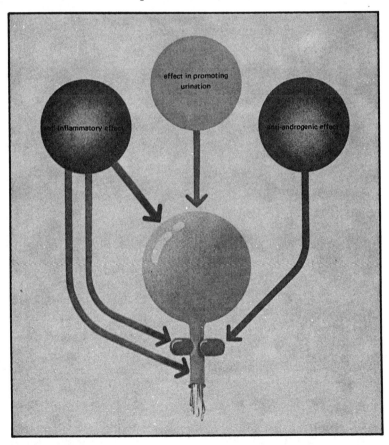

A There is an effect in improving the various symptoms of diseases of the prostate due to the pharmacological action of promoting urination, anti-androgenic hormone and anti-inflammation.

Q. 3   Why should Flower Pollen Extract be effective on dysuria due to diseases of the prostate?

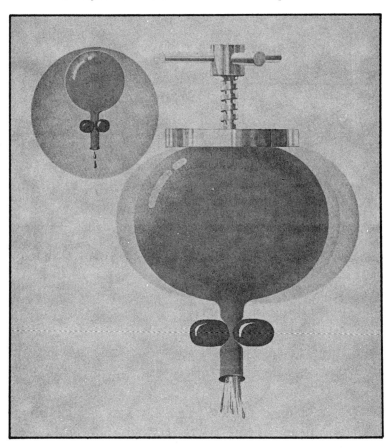

A Measurements of urinary bladder pressure, electromyograms etc. have clearly shown that the contractile power of the urinary bladder is increased in dysuria (due to mechanical pressure resulting from inflammation and hypertrophy of prostate gland).

Q. 4 How does the effect of Flower Pollen Extract in promoting urination differ from that of other drugs?

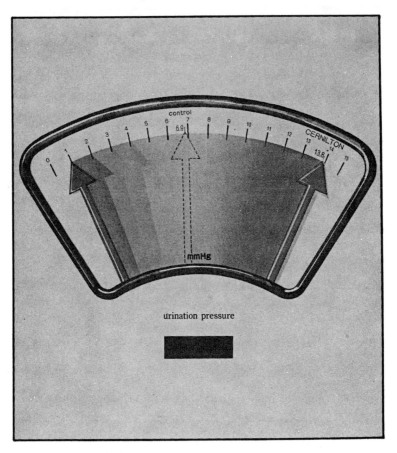

A A study was made of the effect in promoting urination by urination pressure P in animal experiments. The high value of 13.8 mmHg was shown in the group given Flower Pollen Extract orally for 14 days, compared with 6.9 mmHg in the control group, and a higher urination pressure was shown than with other drugs E and D.

Q. 5 **What is meant by the anti-androgenic effect of Flower Pollen Extract?**

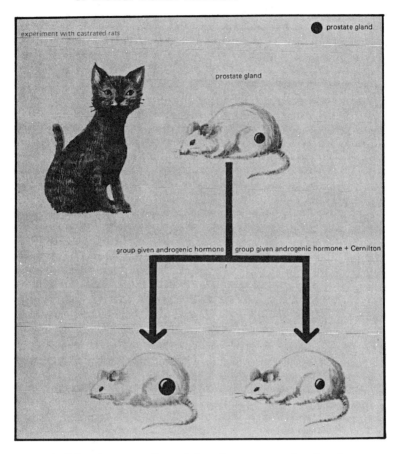

A It has been confirmed that the prostate gland and its hypertrophic portion are dependent on androgenic hormone, and that Flower Pollen Extract acts specifically on the prostate gland, with antagonism to the androgenic hormone (Shida et al., Gunma University.)

Q. 6 What is the difference between the effect of Flower Pollen Extract and that of "E-Drug" on the prostate?

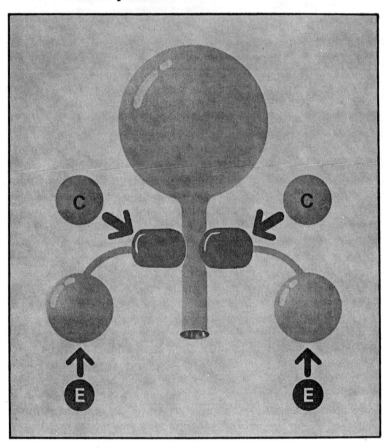

A Both of these drugs have an anti-androgenic action, but it has been confirmed that Flower Pollen Extract acts directly on the prostate gland whereas E-Drug depends on supressing the secretion of androgenic hormone in the testicles.

Q. 7 Why does Flower Pollen Extract have an effect on chronic prostatitis?

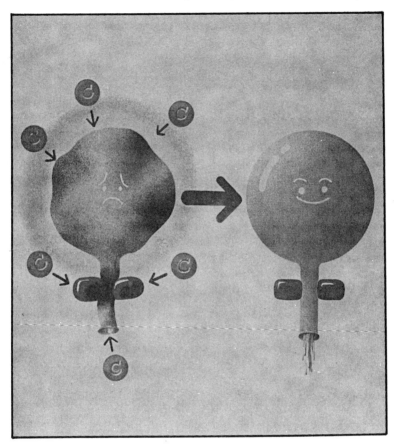

A Flower Pollen Extract increases the resistance of live tissue in the body and exerts an anti-inflammatory effect.

This is shown by its anti-inflammatory action against ovalbumin oedema in the filter paper pellet method, and clinically is observed as disappearance of bacteria from the prostatic fluid and urine.

Q. 8 Are only men suitable subjects for Flower Pollen Extract?

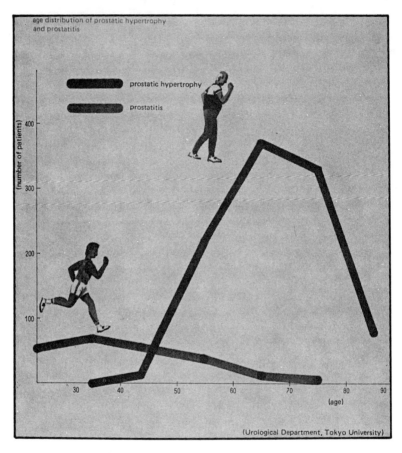

age distribution of prostatic hypertrophy and prostatitis

prostatic hypertrophy

prostatitis

(number of patients)

400

300

200

100

30 40 50 60 70 80 90

(age)

(Urological Department, Tokyo University)

A Chronic prostatitis is also observed in young persons, and there have been more and more cases of prostatic hypertrophy from the late forties onwards. Therefore, Flower Pollen Extract is indicated for dysuria due to diseases of the prostate in both young and old.

Q.9 How does the prostate work?

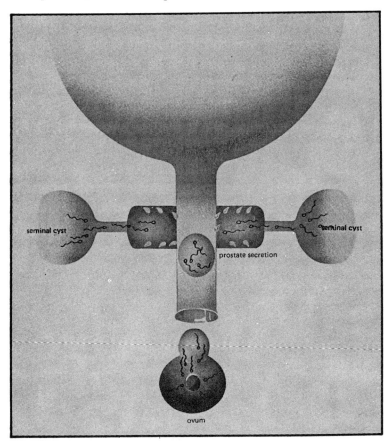

seminal cyst
seminal cyst
prostate secretion
ovum

A It is the glandular tissue which secretes the prostate fluid and accounts for 13-30% of the semen. It is thought to be important chiefly for the fusion of sperm and ovum.

Q. 10   What kind of illness is prostatic hypertrophy?

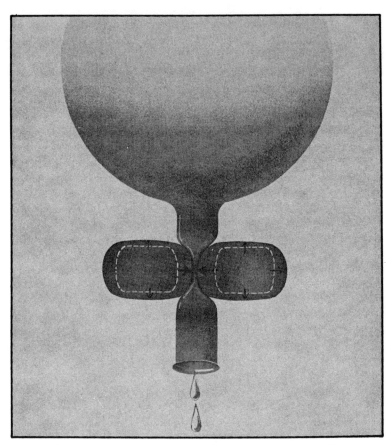

A It is hyperplasia of benign tumor tissue which begins inside the gland in early old age in males (fifties and sixties), gradually compresses the urethra and causes difficulties in urination.

Q. 11 What is the clinical effect of Flower Pollen Extract on chronic prostatitis?

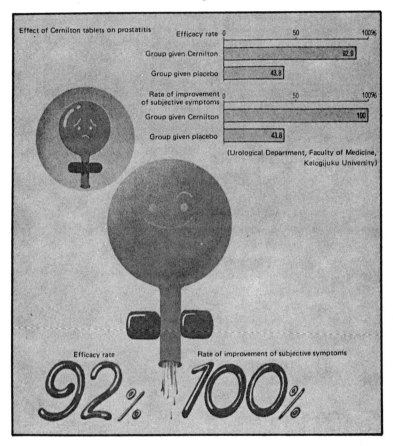

A The effect on chronic prostatitis was studied by the double blind method, using a placebo. The results obtained were for the overall assessment of Flower Pollen Extract: efficacy rate 92.9%, rate of improvement of subjective symptoms 100%, i.e. excellent results.

Q. 12 What is the clinical effect of Flower Pollen Extract on prostatic hypertrophy?

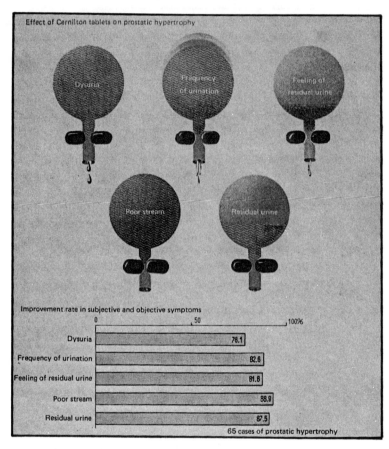

Effect of Cernilton tablets on prostatic hypertrophy

Improvement rate in subjective and objective symptoms

	0	50	100%
Dysuria		78.1	
Frequency of urination		82.6	
Feeling of residual urine		81.8	
Poor stream		88.9	
Residual urine		87.5	

65 cases of prostatic hypertrophy

A Viewing the effectiveness of Flower Pollen Extract on prostatic hypertrophy in the light of subjective and objective symptoms such as dysuria, frequency of urination, residual urine, anuria, etc., in 65 patients in 4 institutions, an excellent rate of improvement of about 80% was shown against all symptoms.

Q. 13 **What is the effect of Flower Pollen Extract on residual urine?**

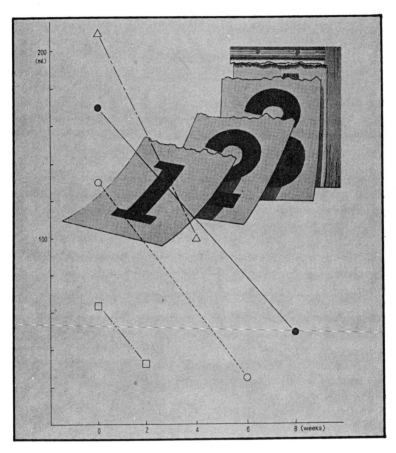

A It is clear from the above diagram that this drug is also effective in reducing residual urine. Even when the amount of residual urine is large, success is achieved by prolonged administration.

Royal Jelly

Another natural product found to aid prostate sufferers is *Royal Jelly*, another gift of the honeybee. *Royal Jelly* is manufactured in the hive for the sole consumption of the queen bee, whose lifespan sometimes surpasses five years. (Worker bees typically live only three to five weeks.)

Royal Jelly is widely known as a dietary supplement, and medical research has confirmed its helpfulness in regulating blood pressure, enhancing the immune system and easing arteriosclerosis and coronary deficiency. Rich in hormones, enzymes, vitamins and amino acids like acetylcholine, *Royal Jelly* is thought to revitalize living cells. The first few doses sometimes produce a characteristic euphoria, which leads some to over-exert themselves.

Two other components of *Royal Jelly* are *gamma globulin* — one of the body's natural antibiotics — and *proteic gelatin,* which builds up the collagen in connective tissues. Soviet scientists found the jelly stimulates the nervous system and speeds glandular secretions, which may explain its reputation as an aphrodisiac.

Elena Groth, a naturopathic physician from Germany, has for years studied the effects of natural medicine on prostate complaints. The most remarkable cases include prostate-related sexual dysfunction - men who could not achieve an erection because of prostate symptoms. After a prescriptive dose of *Royal Jelly*, the majority of Groth's patients report a relief from burning urination and a return of potency in lovemaking.

The use of *Royal Jelly* in prostate cases was discussed at length at a recent convention of English and European urologists. Research continues into how and why this substance works even on advanced cases of *prostatitis* and BPH.

Groth usually prescribes two *Royal Jelly* capsules three times a day, taken along with *flower pollen extract* and a special *seven-herbal tea* — a drink discussed in the following chapter.

Kombucha

Another alternative treatment from Europe is now available in North America. It is a tea-type drink, fermented from the *Kombucha* plant indigenous to Eastern Europe. It works by enhancing the body's metabolism and immune system, and is used throughout the Continent for kidney, liver and gallbladder problems, gout, migraine headaches, rheumatism, arthritis and more.

Dr. Rudolf Sklenar, a German medical doctor, popularized the drink after he noticed the robust health of many elderly Eastern European and Russian peasants. The men boasted of their lovemaking prowess well into their nineties. Sklenar found all these peasants regularly drank *Kombucha* tonic, traditionally believed to have a magical ability to retard male aging.

Sklenar prescribed three cups of *Kombucha* tea per day to a 48-year-old patient who saw it as his last resort before prostate surgery. After two weeks of the treatment, the patient reported increased urine flow and less burning when he urinated. After a month, the man regained his potency and was able to make love to his wife. All without surgery.

Kombucha has been found particularly effective in treating *impotency* in men with *prostate problems*, and those whose sexual problem stems from high blood-pressure medication.

Dozens of other plants have been found to have beneficial effects on men with *prostate problems*. Their functions and uses are detailed in the following chapter.

Chapter 5

Herbal Help for Prostates

We Americans usually turn up our noses at any cure not produced by high technology. We'll gladly swallow the foul-tasting, high-priced cough syrup prescribed by our doctors, but wouldn't think of sipping tea made from an herb in the back yard. Even if it was proven to eliminate coughs.

We have faith in modern medicine. We look to science for answers to life's questions. And while there is no doubt that science and technology have lengthened our lives and spared us countless diseases, we still tend to ignore - or laugh at - non-technological means of solving medical problems. Our open minds slam shut when talk of herbal cures comes up. Words like "poultice" and "elixir" conjure up visions of witch doctors, pipe-smoking grannies or Wild West "Snake Oil" peddlers.

As a society, we don't possess the rich history of natural remedies that is common to Europe. At one time, each village there had its herbalist - someone who knew what plants bring down childhood fevers and which tea helps bruises to heal.

Today, many Americans are more open-minded about herbal medicine. Prostate sufferers may also find relief in "nature's pharmacy." What follows is a listing of "prostate-friendly" herbs and compounds formulated from natural sources.

I am not, by any means, suggesting that herbs alone should be used to treat *prostatitis* or *prostatic hypertrophy*. I propose a marriage of modern and folk remedies. Herbs can be wonderful aids when used in conjunction with modern therapies.

The Small-Flowered Willow Herb

The most potent herb for prostate troubles is an obscure one. So few herbalists wrote of it over the centuries it was almost "lost in time." It is the *small-flowered willow herb*, a water-loving plant that produces tiny white, pink or rust-colored flowers.

Maria Treben, an Austrian herbalist, frequently prescribes a tea made from the herb to men whose prostate problems have laid them low.

"I beg you to show me a way back to health," a German gentleman wrote to Treben. "Give my family back their healthy father."

The man had suffered for years from *chronic prostatitis*. Medications prescribed by his doctor had left him with an ulcer and liver disorders, and still the man passed pus and blood in his stool. The man underwent a prostate surgery with little effect. Additional medications and injections only worsened his condition. Finally, the man turned in despair to the herbalist.

Treben recommended he drink tea made from the *small-flowered willow herb*. Progress was slow at first, but within months his prostate inflammation was relieved. Even the liver disorder and ulcer cleared up.

Another man wrote to Treben to praise the lowly herb. While he was hospitalized with a heart attack, the doctors found he also had a serious *prostate problem*. His medical condition ruled out an operation. The man read in a hospital pamphlet about the *small-flowered willow herb*, and decided he had nothing to lose in trying it.

"I began to drink three cups daily," he wrote. "After several days, I had no more complaints. I still drink two cups a day to ensure a complete recovery. I thank God from the bottom of my heart for the *small-flower willow herb*. It is amazing that medicinal plants can give such results."

One case of the herb's effectiveness was termed a miracle by its beneficiary - a man who knows a miracle when he sees one.

Father Hohmann, a Catholic priest, was diagnosed with terminal prostate cancer. His doctor considered his case hopeless, and told the priest to make his peace and retire. But Father Hohmann wasn't ready to die. A local herbalist prescribed *small-flowered willow herb* tea. And according to the clergyman, his cure was "nothing less than a miracle."

INSTRUCTIONS
Small-flowered Willow Herb Tea

Preparation: Use only the fresh herb, and use the entire plant - stem, leaves and flowers. Mince them finely. Place a heaping teaspoon of the herb in 6 ounces of freshly boiled water. Cover and steep for 3 to 4 minutes; sip hot and unsweetened.

Frequency: One cup twice daily; one before breakfast and one in the evening at least 30 minutes before the final meal of the day.

Where to find Herbal Products

It isn't practical for everyone to cultivate herbs and spend the time mashing up plants to make tea. Happily, there are many very effective herbal-based products on the market aimed at relieving prostate complaints. One of these, mentioned earlier, is *Seven Herbal Tea* — a brew-it-yourself mixture that is available through health food catalogs and stores.

"Seven Herbal Tea" contains *small-flowered willow herb* as well as six other natural plant products known to relieve prostate symptoms, including: *horsetail*, a diuretic and pain reliever; *sage*, an internal cleanser and glandular stimulant; and *saw palmetto*, an herb known to revive atrophied testes. (More about each of these herbs later on.)

This potent tea uses the same formula prescribed by Groth to hundreds of prostate sufferers in Europe. The tea's ability to help even cases declared hopeless accounts for its popularity. It is even credited in part with Europe's statistically lower number of prostate surgeries. It is licensed for sale in the United States.

"Seven Herbal Tea" is sold in loose tea form, because breaking the tea leaves releases essential oils and weakens the effectiveness of the herb.

For those who desire the full Groth therapy for prostate problems, *Flower Pollen Extract* tablets are now available at health food stores. They work in conjunction with the *"Seven Herbal Tea"* to bring relief to the toughest prostate complaints.

Other Herbs

Damiana

Herbalists also attest to the effects of *Damiana*, an herb known as a stimulant in sexual weakness and an overall nerve tonic. In the earlier part of this century, American physician W.H. Myers used *Damiana* extensively in his practice to treat impotency. "I find that in cases of partial impotence and other sexual debility, damiana's success is universal," he wrote. Also Steinmetz of Holland attests to the effect of *Damiana*, and had excellent results with his patients.

INSTRUCTIONS
Damiana Tea

Preparation: Place 2 tablespoons of dried damiana in a cup. Add hot water and let steep for 3 to 5 minutes. Strain and drink hot.

Frequency: One cup daily. **Do not overuse, as liver damage may result.**

Ginseng

Probably the best-known of the so-called aphrodisiac herbs is *ginseng*, otherwise called "man-root." Available as a tea, extract, powder, liquid, capsule or tablet, the pharmacopeia credits *ginseng* with stimulation of androgen production, which assists in sex gland functions. Magical and medicinal properties have been attached to this root for hundreds of years.

Dr. George Zofchak, an herbalist and naturopath from central Pennsylvania, gives detailed advice on the uses of herbs in Mark Bricklin's *Practical Encyclopedia of Natural Healing*. He attests to the usefulness of *Damiana*, and has witnessed *ginseng's* powers as a general normalizing tonic for sexual function.

"*Ginseng* is not going to perform miracles... a cup of *ginseng tea* is not going to abolish a problem that stems from a deep psychological cause," Zofchak said. "But taken over a period of time, ginseng can have a general stimulating and normalizing effect, which may also help the sexual problem."

Zofchak recommends using *ginseng* grown in the United States, which is gathered from mountain areas where it grows wild. Other herbalists prefer Korean or Chinese-grown *ginseng*.

Golden Seal

A tea made from the herb *Golden Seal* is an excellent aid for those with inflammation of the *prostate, colon* and *rectum* - even if the taste is bitter and strong. It is useful, too, for treating *hair loss* and *athlete's foot* infections when a weak solution is applied to the affected area.

INSTRUCTIONS
Golden Seal Tea

Preparation: Steep 1 teaspoon dried Golden Seal root in 1 cup of boiling water for 3 minutes. Strain and sip hot. Tea may be sweetened with honey.

Frequency: several cups, taken throughout the day. **Golden Seal should NOT be used by pregnant women.**

Mallow

Mallow is an herb that provides nourishment to body tissues. It has a prestigious history dating back to Old Testament times. In Job 30:4, the herb is mentioned as one of the few nourishments for people in times of famine.

Cold *mallow tea* could indeed help nourish an ill prostate. It is an excellent aid in cases of *bladder, stomach* and *intestinal inflammation.*

INSTRUCTIONS
Mallow Tea

Preparation: Soak 5 heaping teaspoons of the herb in 2 1/2 quarts of water overnight. In the morning, strain and warm slightly before drinking, but do not boil.

Frequency: Drink 4 cups throughout the day.

Note: It is extremely important that mallow not be heated, as heat destroys its potent qualities.

Herbs That Aid In Urination

Several herbal teas "specialize" in easing painful or difficult urination - a primary symptom of *prostatitis* or BPH. Try several to find the tea that best suits your particular needs and tastes.

Club Moss

This mossy deep-woods trailing plant can aid in easing *inflammation of the testes* as well as *difficult urination*.

INSTRUCTIONS
Club Moss Tea

Preparation: Pour 1 pint of boiling water over 1 level teaspoon Club Moss. Steep for 5 minutes and drain.

Frequency: Drink only one cup daily on an empty stomach - best if used a half hour before breakfast.

Horsetail

The *horsetail herb* is fairly common, growing wild in fields and meadows. It has no leaves or branches. Its shape resembles a slender pine tree, but it seldom grows taller than 10 inches. Sipping a cup of *horsetail tea* - with a little honey, if you wish - may *promote urination*.

INSTRUCTIONS
Horsetail Tea

Preparation: Pour 6 ounces of freshly-boiled water over 1 heaping teaspoon of herb. Cover and steep for 4 to 5 minutes. Strain and sip hot.

Frequency: Use one cup daily.

Wild Thyme

Wild Thyme can grow just about anywhere and likes lots of sun and heat. Its blossoms are small and deep purple, and are a well-known diuretic.

INSTRUCTIONS
Wild Thyme Tea

Preparation: Pour 6 ounces of freshly-boiled water over 1 heaping teaspoon of wild thyme, either fresh or dried. Cover and steep for 3 or 4 minutes. Strain and sweeten with honey.

Frequency: Drink one cup daily.

Stinging Nettle

Don't be intimidated by the mention of *stinging nettles* in the same breath as your urinary equipment. As daunting as it sounds, this 10-inch plant provides soothing *relief to suppressed urination and inflamed urinary tracts.*

The plant has drooping heart-shaped leaves and is covered with protective "stinging" hairs. If you pick it fresh, make sure to wear gloves.

INSTRUCTIONS
Stinging Nettle Tea

Preparation: Pour 6 ounces of freshly boiled water over 1 heaping teaspoon of the herb. Cover, steep for 3 minutes. Strain and sip unsweetened.

Frequency: Sip several cups throughout the day. Do not sweeten. If you find the tea bitter, add a little chamomile or mint to the boiling water mix.

Greater Celandine

Greater Celandine, a slender, many-branched herb with a soft hairy covering, aids in *easing painful urination* - another common prostate symptom. It is also an excellent *aid to liver problems.*

Greater Celandine Tea

Preparation: Pour 1 pint freshly boiled water over 2 level teaspoons of the herb. Strain and sip. Honey may be added.

Frequency: Drink several cups throughout the day.

Other helpful herbs

Dr. Zofchak likes to blend his own tea for urinary problems: a mixture of *buchu leaves* (a bladder soother), *bearberry* (also called uva-ursi), *cubeb berries* and *mallow.* He adds *anise* and *licorice* for taste and "balance."

An herb called *St. Johnswort* is useful in urinary incontinence, Zofchak said.

Zofchak's prostate cures include teas made from *buchu leaves, uva-ursi and saw palmetto.*

A Word of Caution

Some doctors do not believe in herbal therapies for diseases, and caution patients against their use. Most doctors are not trained in the helpful uses and cures brought about by nature, and are very cautious about even new technological "cure-alls."

Doctors are correct in their caution. Indeed, many herbs are beneficial when used in carefully controlled doses, while overuse or incorrect handling can result in poisoning.

As Bricklin says in his *Encyclopedia of Natural Healing*, never take any herb unless you know exactly what it is and what it may do.

Chapter 6

Diet As A Cure and Preventive

What goes into your body in a big way determines what comes out: good health, vigor and long life, or chronic illness, listlessness and a shortened lifespan. Many physicians of different specialties have devised diet plans to suit almost every physical need. Prostate sufferers are no different.

Homeostasis and Diet

Dr. Jonn Matsen, a Canadian naturopathic doctor and author, believes that not all sickness is caused by outside forces attacking body cells. He teaches that certain types of food can trigger bodily dysfunctions - including *prostatitis* and *prostatic hypertrophy*.

Matsen views the body as one cooperative unit. *Homeostasis* is a state of perfect bodily regulation, when all the body's cells work together as one. (This bodily philosophy can be found in ancient Eastern disciplines like Tao, Zen and Hinduism.) When acute disease strikes - occasional bouts of sickness that come and go quickly - It may be the body attempting to re-establish *homeostasis* after it has been abused, Matsen says.

The doctor says part of the American male's prostate problem is the endless variety of processed and "junk" foods the average person eats from childhood. Eating these foods shocks the digestive system, which was not designed to break down the complex chemicals added as preservatives, flavor enhancers of coloring agents.

A body can handle an occasional dose of snack cakes and potato chips, but a regular diet of them can produce an overabundance of intestinal toxins. These overload the body's capacity to process food. Its energies go toward ridding itself of toxins rather than performing its intended task: absorbing nutrients vital to good health.

In order to rid patients of years of built-up toxins, Matsen devised a rigorous diet that hundreds of patients say brought them out of lives of fatigue and illness and back to robust health.

Starting the diet is the hardest step: permanently eliminating American staples like chocolate, coffee, tea, refined sugar, artificial sweeteners, preservatives, salt and alcohol.

Depending on the dieter's medical needs, he next temporarily gives up certain groups of foods for several weeks. These may include peanuts, yeast, pork, shellfish, turkey, chicken, carrots, strawberries, cucumbers, walnuts and maple syrup.

These foods are gradually re-introduced to the diet after several weeks, after the body has regained its ability to properly process food - the most important step to regaining *homeostasis*.

One of Matsen's most enthusiastic patients suffered from a colonic polyp - a growth in his lower bowel. He was overweight, suffered from high blood pressure and suffered from frequent bouts of painful abdominal gas.

After six months on Matsen's detoxification diet, the man's weight and blood pressure were down to healthy levels. His abdominal gas pain had almost disappeared.

Those interested in learning more about the *homeostasis* diet can read Matsen's best-selling book *The Mysterious Cause of Illness and How to Overcome Every Disease from Constipation to Cancer.* (Available from Fischer Publishing, Canfield, OH).

Avoidance Tactics

Many doctors agree that men with prostate problems may want to avoid certain types of foods - they either interfere with medications, irritate swollen tissues, promote urination or are linked with androgen, cholesterol or carcinogen production.

In chapter 3, I covered the effects of fat, cholesterol, zinc and several other dietary items on prostate health. To recap those points, Dr. Peter Hill of the American Health Foundation in New York City said "...by reducing total calorie intake, and substituting fruit and vegetable calories for animal calories, a high-risk prostatic cancer group was switched to a low-risk one."

Red meat has its downside. Although it is a great source of protein, it must be prepared just the right way to keep its negative effects from outweighing its benefits. Fatty cuts and most pork selections should be avoided, or at least carefully trimmed of excess fat before cooking.

Care should be taken while grilling meat: charcoal by-products and charring have been linked with cancer. Say no to the popular Cajun practice of "blackening" meats. Also, any meat preserved with nitrites - like bacon, cold cuts, sausage or smoked chops - should be avoided. Nitrites are carcinogens (cancer-linked chemicals), and are known to irritate enlarged glands.

Other items to avoid include tomato-based food, chocolate, caffeine, pickled foods, margarine and processed foods. Alcohol is very irritating to prostate tissue, and some men react to the flavorings in certain drinks with a type of chronic prostatitis. It's important to get enough oil in the diet, but stick to olive or safflower oils, and use them sparingly. Although *unrefined flaxseed* and *pumpkin seed oils* are recommended throughout this book, *use them only on salads* - heating them drives off their beneficial contents.

Consider Positive Foods

Instead of mulling over what you CAN'T eat, consider all the fine things you can enjoy on a sensible diet. Eat at least one large salad each day, and let its production be an outlet for your culinary creativity. By mixing colors, shapes and shades of vegetables, fruits, nuts and sprouts, you can enjoy your meal with all five of your senses.

One advantage to salads is their high fiber content. Researchers believe that a diet with lots of beans, fruit, and whole-wheat bread can further lower prostate risks. Men who eat more fiber get less prostate cancer, too.

Instead of eating dessert, have a piece of fresh fruit after your meal. If it is possible, stay out of the kitchen when you aren't there for a meal. Remove the salt shaker and sugar bowl from the table, so you won't be tempted. Shop for groceries *after* you've had a filling meal, so those "junk" items won't seem so appealing. Buy fresh "whole" foods whenever possible: nutritionists say that a fresh orange or grape is twice as good for you as the juice, especially if you're trying to keep your weight under control.

As Bricklin suggests in his *Encyclopedia*, double your buying in the store's produce section, and halve your meat and deli purchases. Your prostate - and the rest of your body - will thank you.

Most people find they feel the effects of an improved diet only days after changing their eating habits. They feel more energetic and less moody, and the usual aches and pains simply don't occupy them as much. Add to this the all-important element of prevention: study after study links a low-fat, sensible diet to a decrease in cancer risk. Those already diagnosed with cancer can use natural methods to alleviate their symptoms and sometimes even send the disease into remission - these concepts are covered in a later chapter.

But like the old saying goes: an ounce of prevention is worth a pound of cure. The United States Department of Agriculture in 1993 released a new "food pyramid" system to measure the types and amounts of foods important to daily diets. Their recommendations are reprinted on the following pages.

Food Guide Pyramid
A Guide to Daily Food Choices

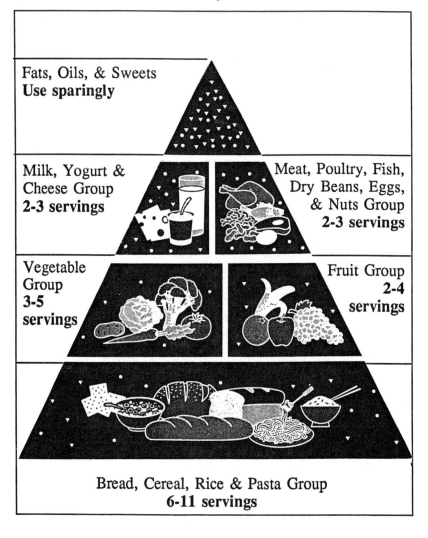

Fats, Oils, & Sweets
Use sparingly

Milk, Yogurt &
Cheese Group
2-3 servings

Meat, Poultry, Fish,
Dry Beans, Eggs,
& Nuts Group
2-3 servings

Vegetable
Group
**3-5
servings**

Fruit Group
**2-4
servings**

Bread, Cereal, Rice & Pasta Group
6-11 servings

KEY- These symbols show fats, oil, and added sugars in foods.

◘ Fat (naturally occuring and added)

▲ Sugars (added)

How many servings do you need each day?

	Women & some older adults	Children teen girls active women, most men	Teen boys & active men
Bread group	6	9	11
Vegetable group	3	4	5
Fruit group	2	3	4
Milk group	2-3*	2-3*	2-3*
Meat group	2	2	3

*Women who are pregnant or breastfeeding, teenagers, and young adults to age 24 need 3 servings.

What counts as one serving?

Breads, Cereals, Rice, Pasta
1 slice of bread
1/2 cup of cooked cereal, rice, or pasta
1 ounce of dry cereal

Fruits
1 medium whole fruit
3/4 cup of juice
1/2 cup of canned fruit

Vegetables
1/2 cup cooked vegetables
1 cup of tossed salad

Milk
1 cup of milk
8 ounces of yogurt
1-1/2 to 2 ounces of cheese

Meat, Poultry, Fish, Eggs, Dry Beans, and Nuts
3 ounces of cooked meat, poultry, or fish (3 ounces of meat is about the same size as a deck of cards)

1/2 cup of cooked beans or 2 tablespoons of peanut butter or 1 egg counts the same as 1 ounce of meat (about 1/3 serving)

Fats, Oils, and Sweets
Use sparingly. These are foods such as salad dressings, cream, butter, margarine, sugars, soft drinks and candies. Go easy on these foods because they have a lot of calories from fat and sugars, but few nutrients.

A no-nonsense diet can be boosted by supplemental doses of *amino acids (L-glycine, L-alanine and L-glutamine)*, *B-vitamins, zinc, vitamins A and E* and a little daily dose of *unrefined flaxseed* or *pumpkin seed oil*, which provide essential fatty acids needed for a healthy prostate.

Some nutrition authorities swear by the use of *prostate glandulars* - the use of a raw concentrate of the gland or organ that is problematic. Thus, many prostate-specific vitamin formulations will contain doses of ground bovine prostatic tissue - cow prostate. Some believe these tissues supply prostate-specific nutritional compounds that don't occur anywhere else.

Nutritional Research News supplies a "label check" for men shopping for a prostate supplement at their vitamin store:

Label Check for Prostate Supplements

✓ Extract lipid sterolic serona repens (Saw Palmetto)

✓ Aminoacetic acid

✓ Aminopropionic acid

✓ Alpha-aminoglutaric acid

✓ Raw prostate concentrate

✓ Zinc (glucinate)

✓ Vitamin B6 (Pyridoxine HCl)

✓ Vitamin A (Palmitate)

✓ Vitamin E (D-alpha tocopherol succinate)

✓ Pumpkin seed oil

✓ Cold-pressed, unrefined Flaxseed oil

✓ Ginseng (powder, liquid, tablets, tea, extract, capsules)

Dr. Heinrich Hergut, a Nuremberg physician, wrote an entire book on diet for men with prostate illnesses. Included here are several of the recipes made with ingredients available in markets, co-ops and health food stores in the United States.

Juices and Purees

Raw food, extracted mechanically from the source, supplies rich nutrition - even for those on soft-food and non-cellulose diets.

Unreduced, fresh food is always preferable, however, and can never be completely replaced by juices. As soon as your physician allows, return to fruit and raw vegetables.

Make sure all the produce you use is well washed. Trim off any bruises or spoiled spots. Many juicers and presses are available, from the small hand press to the motorized centerfuge. Hand presses require the fruit to be chopped first. Even when using an electric machine, it's a good idea to grate or chop apples, pears, tubers, leafy vegetables and herbs. Those who cannot prepare juices themselves can find high-quality grape juice, fruit juices and vegetable juices in bottles at the health food store.

Fruit juices:

Always serve fresh-squeezed fruit juice right away. Any delay means loss of food value. The following fruits provide delicious and wholesome juice without any admixture or extra processing:

Oranges, mandarin oranges, tangerines, grapefruit, apples, pears, grapes, strawberries, blueberries, currants, raspberries, peaches, apricots, sweet plums, melons and cherries.

Many juices taste even better when mixed with one another - just check the wide variety of combinations available at the supermarket! It's best to use a citrus fruit as a "base," and add the juice of other, sweeter juices like berry, peach, apricot or plum. For a milkshake-like texture, add a pureed banana; or create a "smoothie" by using fresh, frozen fruit whirled with ice cubes in a blender or food processor.

Other additions and accents include lemon juice, unrefined sugar, honey, fruit concentrate, yogurt, buttermilk, linseed, rice or barley puree.

Vegetable Juices

Pureed vegetables should also be served fresh to preserve vitamins and minerals.

The following vegetables taste fine served alone: tomato, turnip, beet, radish, cabbage, celery and all leafy, tuberous root vegetables.

Our favorite mixed vegetable juice includes equal parts of turnips, tomatoes and spinach. Other vegetables or flavorings may be added to your taste - just avoid too much salt, sugar or restricted items. The following provide tasty alternatives when added to your favorite vegetable juice mix: sorrel, nettle, chives, parsley, onion, tender celery and other herbs.

Try adding the following to your glassful of vegetable juice: a tablespoon of yogurt or buttermilk; lemon juice, fruit juice concentrate, linseed, rice or barley puree. Pureed leafy vegetables are also favored: try white and green cabbage, endive, bok choy, or dandelion. In the springtime, gather up and add some blood-cleansing juices of nettle, sorrel or dandelion.

If you find fresh vegetable juice too bitter or sharp-tasting, try adding a little *rice or barley flour essence.* **To make:** Stir a heaping teaspoon flour into 7 oz. cold water; boil for 5 minutes, stirring constantly. Allow mixture to cool, and add a sprinkling to each glass of vegetable juice you make. Use with care, as too much could prove constipating.

Linseed paste will also take the edge off fresh juice. It has a mildly cathartic effect on the bowels. **To make:** combine 1 tablespoon linseeds in 7 oz. water. Wash, then boil 10 minutes. Sift out the hulls and allow to cool. Prepare a day's supply each morning and keep in a thermos for blending with juices throughout the day.

Soy milk is a high-protein, mild substitute for cow's milk. **To make:** soak 1 cup of soybeans in 7 cups water for two hours. Using the same water, boil for 20 minutes, stirring constantly. Strain juice into a pan. Add water to cow's milk consistency. Add two tablespoons of fruit sugar, let cool.

Meusli: Breakfast of Generations

The original apple meusli cereal, as first introduced by Dr. Bircher, has remained a mainstay of healthy diets through many years of treatment.

The original German recipe calls for sour, fleshy, juicy apples like Jonathan, Granny Smith or Rome, but modern usage includes just about any apple you find satisfying. If late-season apples proved dry or bland, enrich the aroma by adding a little freshly grated orange peel. Some cooks "dress up" their meusli by sprinkling on a little orange juice or rose-hip puree just before serving.

Dr. Bircher's Apple Meusli

1 tablespoon rolled oats, soaked for 12 hours in
3 tablespoons cold water
(If using quick-cooking oats, simply blend together
oats and water)

Add and mix to a smooth consistency:

1 teaspoon lemon juice or orange juice
1 tablespoon plain yogurt
a little honey
1-2 tablespoons water

Wash, stem and core 1/2 lb. apples. Grate the apples directly into the oat mixture, stirring occasionally so the apples do not turn brown. This makes 1 serving.

Serve immediately, garnished with a teaspoon of grated almonds. (Don't use walnuts or hazelnuts - they are too hard to digest.)

Options:

Instead of rolled oats, use a pre-soaked tablespoonful of wheat germ, rice, barley, rye, buckwheat, millet or soy flakes. To add a boost of B-vitamins, add a bit of yeast flakes, available in health food stores.

For those forbidden to consume protein, serve apple meusli with almond or sesame puree: instead of yogurt and lemon juice, use a tablespoon of ground almonds or sesame seeds, and increase added water to 3 tablespoons.

Those with lactose intolerance may try the following recipe. It has a sharper taste and is less filling, but it promotes digestion and protects the liver. It is especially valuable for elderly people because it is high in unsaturated fatty acids.

1 tablespoon rolled oats, soaked
3 tablespoons orange juice
2 tablespoons yogurt
1 tablespoon lowfat cottage cheese
1 tablespoon honey
1 tablespoon linseed oil

Mix together all the above till smooth. Grate in 1 large apple and 1 beaten banana.

Those on a *weight-gain diet* will appreciate their apple meusli with cream. Follow the basic recipe for apple meusli, but beat 3 or 4 tablespoons of cream together with the lemon or orange juice.

For a special treat and an increase in your *Vitamin C intake*, make meusli with berries or small, pit-producing fruits. Don't use any sour berries!

Use 1/2 pound of washed, selected and crushed:

strawberries   blueberries
raspberries   blackberries

Or pitted and finely chopped or food-processed:

plums   peaches
apricots

Add the fruit to the basic Meusli oat or grain mixture, instead of apples.

Try the following fruit combinations, using the same 1/2-pound proportion as the apples in the recipe:

strawberries and raspberries
strawberries and apples
blackberries and apples
apples with finely cut orange or tangerine segments
apples and bananas

Raw Vegetables

Observe the following four principals when preparing raw vegetables:

1. Process Quickly

Sun-ripened, organically grown vegetables are best, preferably grown in your own garden. Raw vegetables should be processed as little as possible and be served immediately, before wilting or loss of juice occurs. When using chopped or cut-up vegetables, serve as soon as possible to limit exposure to air.

2. Buy Quality

Buy leafy and root vegetables that are young and tender, fully colored on all sides and symmetrically shaped. If possible, buy produce that was grown without chemical fertilizers. This is especially important to cooks whose food is served to the ill.

3. Clean Vegetables Properly

To prevent insect infestation and infection from e-coli bacteria, scrub root vegetables under running water with a vegetable brush. If possible, make sure they were grown in a garden that does not use liquified manure or purified plant sludge for fertilizer. Peel and immerse immediately in cold water with a little lemon juice and salt added - this preserves the bright, fresh color.

Leafy vegetables, lettuces and cabbages should be separated from their stems, cleaned of brown or damaged areas and allowed to soak in mildly salted water for 15 minutes - this cleanses the nooks and crannies of hidden worms and insects. Rinse each leaf seperately under running water. Drain well.

Vegetables with smaller leaves, like dandelions, brussels sprouts and spinach should be carefully trimmed of tough stems and rootlets. Process these in small portions.

Tomatoes, cucumbers and peppers - known in Germany as "fruit vegetables," require specialized processing. Cucumbers should be peeled from the center toward the outside. Trim off the ends. Small, tender cucumbers are fine if eaten unpeeled. Use only young peppers for salads. Don't peel these - simply cut them in half and remove the core. Soak peppers in water if they taste bitter.

If there is any doubt about the farm fertilization methods used to grow the vegetables, soak them 15 minutes in a mild salt water solution. The salt water dissolves the protein film that coats the vegetable and gives a foothold to worm eggs and vermin. Any unwelcome "dinner guests " are washed away when the food is subsequently rinsed.

Sterilize tuberous (root) vegetables by immersing the prepared vegetables in boiling water for 10 seconds. This kills germs on the outside, while leaving the insides raw.

Vegetable and fruit juices become virtually germ-free with the addition of squeezed lemon juice.

4. Harmonious Combinations

Every raw vegetable dish should, if possible, contain the "triad:" a root, a fruit and a leafy vegetable. Green leaf is especially important for the ill. Sauces and garnishes can add the variety that relieves dietary boredom.

Neat little trimmings of herbs, radishes, young carrots, etc. can lend the raw vegetable dish a colorful, festive appearance. A serving with at least three colors enhances the beauty of the dish and contributes to the pleasure of eating. Vary combinations throughout the day, but avoid combining more than three vegetables. Try not to be too varied - even variety can get old, and excessive change can be hard on digestion.

Try preparing the following vegetables the European way:

Lettuce, endives	serve whole leaves, or cut largest leaves in half.
Spinach, leeks, peppers stalk celery, fennel	cut into fine strips
Cabbages- white, red and purple	slice leaves finely
Small turnips, celery, beets, radishes	grate in food processor or by hand
Jerusalem artichokes, kohlrabi, cucumber, zucchini, summer squash	slice thin
Cauliflower	cut flower and tender parts of stem into thin slices

Sauces and Dressings for Raw Vegetables

Herb Oil Sauce

1 tablespoon unrefined flaxseed oil
1 teaspoon lemon juice
1 teaspoon minced onion or garlic
1 teaspoon fresh herbs, or 1 pinch dried herbs

Mix together well; use as a dip or pour over vegetable dish before serving.

Mayonnaise Sauce

1 beaten egg yolk
1/2 cup unrefined flaxseed oil

Add the oil a drop at a time to the egg yolk while stirring steadily with a beater. This mixture is enough for six individual portions:

For a single serving, mix together 1 tablespoon of the above yolk-oil mixture; 1 teaspoon lemon juice; a little onion or garlic, minced; and a teaspoon of herbs.

Vegetarian or Vegetable-protein Mayonnaise Sauce

2 tablespoons soy flour
6 tablespoons water

Combine to a smooth batter. Alternately add the following while steadily stirring:

2 teaspoons flaxseed oil
3 tablespoons lemon juice
garlic, onion or herbs to taste

Lowfat Cottage Cheese Dressing

1/2 cup lowfat cottage cheese
1/2 teaspoon lemon juice
buttermilk as needed

Beat together to a thick sauce. Season with a little salt, chives or parsley to taste. Use spinach or carrot juice to vary the color and taste. This is especially good served with fresh artichokes or asparagus. Try it with a raw tomato stuffed with cucumbers, celery, cauliflower or white cabbage.

Yogurt Dip

2-3 tablespoons lowfat yogurt (plain)
several drops lemon juice
a little minced onion or garlic
fresh or dried herbs to taste

Beat ingredients together in a small bowl; serve as a dip.

Almond or Sesame Sauce

1 tablespoon ground almonds or pureed sesame seeds
3 tablespoons water
1 teaspoon lemon juice
onion or garlic, minced
herbs to taste

Add other ingredients slowly to almonds or sesame. This is especially good for those on diets that forbid animal protein.

Carrot Sauce

1 medium-large carrot
2 tablespoons vegetable broth
pinch salt
minced onion or rosemary

Place all ingredients in mixer or food processor and puree.

Vinaigrette

1 tablespoon wheat germ oil
1 teaspoon lemon juice
1 teaspoon water or vegetable broth
1 teaspoon boiled onion
1-2 sweet pickles, chopped fine
1 teaspoon diced tomato

Combine together and season with parsley, chives and a little herbal salt.

Make your own Sprouts

Wheat, rye, barley, mung beans and oats can be found at any feed store, co-op or natural foods outlet. Sprouts made from these grains are a delicious, wholesome addition to any meal or salad.

To sprout your own grain: In the evening, wash about 2 cups of grain in a sieve under a stream of water and place it in a small bowl. Cover with water and place in a warm spot overnight.

The following morning, rinse the grain and spread it out on a plate or cookie sheet to dry. Leave in a warm spot till evening, when you should return it to its bowl and cover it again with water overnight.

Repeat the process the following day. By day 4, your grain will have developed sprouts of 1/4 to 1/2 inch. Snip off what you like. Take a mason jar or other wide-mouth glass vessel and lay a water-soaked paper towel inside. Lay the jar on its side, spread the sprouted grain atop the towel and replace the lid. Keep the jar in a warm place, keep the towel damp, and replace with more sprouted grain when the supply is low. Thus you can keep a good, fresh vegetable and garnish on hand at all times.

Recipes for Cooked Vegetable Dishes

The first consideration when cooking vegetables is fat. For cooking, use only small amounts of sweet (unsalted) butter; sunflower, corn oils and germ oils. Cold-pressed sunflower oil and olive oils are good choices for salads and sauces. They are rich in unsaturated fatty acids. Their purity makes them more easily digested than many other oils. Just remember not to heat them too quickly or intensely, as they will burn!

Soups: Recipes for One

We use quite a lot of vegetable broth in our recipes, but in a small household, fresh vegetable broth cannot be prepared every day. Instead, try using ordinary tap water and an added seasoning like yeast extract (a good source of B vitamins) or vegetable buillion. A little cream or milk improves every soup and vegetable.

Vegetable Broth

> 1 tablespoon butter
> 1 onion, halved
> 1 stalk celery
> endive
> cabbage
> 1 stalk leek

Cut the vegetables into small pieces and steam for at least 15 minutes over low heat.

Add vegetables and butter to 2 quarts cold water. Bring to boil, reduce heat and simmer for two hours. Season mildly with lovage or other herbs, 1/2 bay leaf and a pinch of salt.

Pour through a sieve and serve as a clear broth.

Clear Rice Soup

> 1/2 tablespoon butter
> a little chopped onion
> a little celery and leek, cut fine
> 2 cups vegetable broth
> 1 tablespoon unpolished rice
> 1 pinch salt

Steam all ingredients together for 45 minutes over low heat. Sieve and serve as clear broth.

For a thicker, more filling soup, sprinkle 1/2 tablespoon whole wheat or buckwheat flour over the steamed mixture. Add 1 cup of vegetable broth or water, and boil another 30 minutes. Add 1/2 tablespoon milk and chopped chives to tureen before serving. May also be seasoned with marjoram, nutmeg or caraway.

Herb Soup

 1 tablespoon whole wheat flour
 1/2 cup milk
 5 cups vegetable broth, boiling

Mix the flour into half the milk and stir into the boiling broth. Simmer for 15 minutes.

Mix a tablespoon of soy flour with the remaining milk and put into the soup tureen. Beat the mixture with a hand mixer. Season with pinches of salt, lovage, marjoram, chives, nutmeg or caraway.

Soy Soup

 1/2 tablespoon butter
 a little chopped onion, steamed
 1 tablespoon whole wheat flour
 1/2 tablespoon soy flour
 1/2 tomato, peeled and diced (add just before serving)

Season with a pinch of salt, rosemary, chives and parsley.

Oat Cream Soup

 1/2 tablespoon flour, toasted lightly in a skillet
 2 tablespoons rolled oats
 3 cups vegetable broth
 a little celery

Combine ingredients and simmer 1 hour; strain. Add a tablespoon of butter to the tureen. Season with a pinch of salt; yeast extract, chives, or rosemary.

Kale Soup

1/2 tablespoon butter
a little onion, chopped and steamed briefly
1 tablespoon leek, chopped
1 stalk celery, diced
1 large leaf of kale, soaked 12 hours in a quart of water
1 cup water
5 cups vegetable broth

Mix together in saucepan and simmer 60 to 90 minutes. Season with celery seed, salt or ground pepper.

Tomato Soup 1

1/2 tablespoon butter
a little onion
2 tablespoons small turnips
celery
leek
1 clove garlic
a little rosemary

Cut everything finely together and steam for 10 minutes.
Add 1 tomato, chopped
Sprinkle with 1 tablespoon whole wheat flour

Add 3 cups vegetable broth. Simmer for 30 minutes, strain and serve. Season with salt, cloves, chives, bay leaf. Also good with 1/4 cup steamed rice added.

Tomato Soup 2

4 ripe summer tomatoes, cut up, boiled and strained
1 teaspoon lemon juice or fructose

Add one cup milk or buttermilk. Mix well; serve lukewarm or cold.

Potato Soup with Leeks

1/2 tablespoon butter
1/2 leek, cut in strips and steamed well
1/2 teaspoon whole wheat flour, sprinkled over leeks
 and butter
3 cups vegetable broth, boiling

Combine the above. Cut in 1 medium potato and boil until it is soft. Season with a pinch of salt, yeast extract and marjoram.

Minestrone

1/2 tablespoon butter
a little onion, steamed together with
2 tablespoons leek, cut fine, and
a few celery leaves
1 cup endive leaves

Combine in 4 cups of vegetable broth, season with salt, parsley and chives, and simmer for 30 minutes. Add 1 teaspoon thyme, 1/2 clove garlic, 1/2 cup whole-grain pasta or brown rice. Simmer together for 15 to 20 minutes. Enhance with a small pat of butter.

Sandwiches

Sandwiches are popular the world over. Served as an hors d'oeuvre for evening meals or as ready lunches on the road, this quick and easy food comes in endless variations. Men with prostate problems are usually told to stick with thin-sliced, whole-grain breads. Included here are recipes for spreads and suggested ingredients that can be arranged in all sorts of combinations to create an attractive, fresh and appetizing appearance.

Basic Sandwich Spread

lowfat cottage cheese or butter, stirred until frothy, a little yeast extract, mixed in chives, herbs, caraway seeds or tomato puree, according to taste.

Dress up spread sandwiches with :

carrots	onions cut in rings
raw celery	capers
tomatoes	olives
radishes	lettuces
water cress	

Boiled and Steamed Vegetables

Boiled vegetables are mild on digestion but pack plenty of vitamins. Men recovering from surgery, radiation or chemotherapy treatments are advised to read the following carefully and put the recipes to use to ensure a quick recovery.

It is important that little salt be used to prepare all these dishes. Judicious use of spices and herbs can largely replace salt - but beware of supermarket "salt substitutes." These frequently contain preservatives and flavor enhancers that could be more damaging than the real thing!

Most boiled vegetables should be served "au naturel" - that is, without dressing-up or garnishing. Endive, fennel, carrots, tomatoes, zucchini, beets, eggplant and artichokes are especially good prepared this way. Avoid gas-producers like cabbage, peas, beans and spinach until your digestive system is fully recovered from your treatment or surgery.

Preparation is easy: simply steam vegetables in or over a pan of vegetable broth or water until they are soft. Cut the vegetables into smaller pieces according to its variety.

Serve with butter, if you must, or sprinkle with herbs. Two special vegetables are artichokes and corn on the cob:

Artichokes

Cut the stems off one or two artichokes, up close to the heads. Remove the undermost, hard leaves, cut off the leaf tips. Halve the heads and cut out the blossoms. Wash in running water. Put 1/2 teaspoon lemon juice on the cut halves. Lay the artichokes in 2 cups water. Bring to boil and simmer 45 minutes, until artichokes are soft. Drain. Serve on a warm dish, covered with a napkin. Very good served with cottage cheese sauce or vinaigrette.

Corn on the Cob

Take one or two ears of fresh corn, shucks and silk removed. Drop them in a pan of boiling, salted water and cook for 10 minutes. Serve with fresh butter or lowfat cottage cheese. Be sure to chew each bite well or the corn will not properly digest.

Stalk Celery

Cut 3 or 4 stalks of celery into 3-inch pieces

Steam briefly in a frying pan

In the meantime, combine

1/2 onion, chopped
1 cup vegetable broth
2 tablespoons milk or a little lemon juice
a pinch of salt

Simmer together until tender, about 30 minutes. Combine with celery stalks in frying pan; season with celery seed and yeast extract.

Steamed Celery

1/2 tablespoon butter

1/2 onion, steamed briefly

3 or 4 stalks celery with tops, cut into small slices
and steamed

Add 2 cups of vegetable broth, simmer 30 - 45 minutes until celery is tender. Season with marjoram or lemon juice.

Celery Sections

1 stalk celery,

Cut celery into quarters and boil until tender in:

1/2 cup milk

1/2 cup water

pinch of salt

Cut into wafer-thin slices and serve like flakes on a hot serving plate. Cover with toasted cracker crumbs and melted butter.

Chopped Spinach

Carefully select four to six deep-green spinach leaves. Chop them up; discard any thick stems; wash well. Boil briskly a short while in 2 cups of vegetable broth. Reserve broth.

In a seperate container, steam together briefly

a little chopped onion

a little garlic

Remove from heat. Add:

1 tablespoon flour

the water poured off the spinach, above

a pinch of salt

Simmer all together for 15 minutes. Add the spinach and heat through. Season with peppermint leaves, sage and fresh butter.

Just before serving, add 1 cup finely chopped raw spinach leaves.

*Do not serve spinach to patients with diarrhea.

Green Peas

    1/2 tablespoon butter
    a little onion, lightly steamed
    3/4 cup green peas
    1 cup vegetable broth
    pinch of salt.

Combine ingredients in frying pan; boil for 10 minutes. Season with parsley, chives or marjoram.

*Peas should be served only to those who can tolerate them. Do not serve them to patients plagued with flatulence!

Red Beets

Simmer 2 cups red beets for two hours. Peel and cut into thin slices. Melt 1/2 tablespoon butter and add to the beets. Pour in 1/2 cup vegetable broth and steam for 15 minutes. Add a pinch of salt and 1/2 tablespoon flour before serving. Season with lemon, caraway, lemon balm, nutmeg, parsley or a little garlic.

Stewed Tomatoes

Blanch 4 or 5 fresh tomatoes in boiling water, peel. Place in frying pan with a tablespoon of oil, 1/2 tablespoon butter, 1/2 onion. and a sprinkling of fruit sugar. Steam together, breaking up tomatoes as they cook and thicken. Add a little minced garlic and a tablespoon of cornstarch for binding; then a pinch of chopped parsley. Other herbs like rosemary, basil, chives or marjoram may be sprinkled over the tomatoes when they are served.

Stuffed Tomatoes

Cut the tops off two or three tomatoes. Hollow them out, chop the pulp and mix with 1 teaspoon of uncooked rice per tomato. Replace in the tomato shell. Season to taste with rosemary, basil, onion or garlic. Put 1/2 teaspoon butter atop each, replace the tops. Bake at 325° F for 30 minutes. Sprinkle with toasted crumbs and serve with a cup of soup.

Tomatoes with Scrambled Eggs

1 or two tomatoes, cut up and stewed
1 large egg or 1 portion egg substitute
1 tablespoon cream
pinch of salt

Mix together all ingredients and scramble in small frying pan. Season with chives or garlic.

Red Cabbage

1/2 tablespoon butter
1/2 onion, chopped
2 cups red cabbage, sliced fine

Steam all three ingredients together for 15 minutes. Add:

1/2 tablespoon lemon juice
1/2 apple, sliced thin
1/2 tablespoon rice
1 1/2 cups vegetable broth

Steam all ingredients over low heat for 1 to 1 1/2 hours. Spread on a baking sheet, coat with butter and broil briefly.

Garnish at serving with mixture of 1/2 cup grape juice or fruit juice, a peeled, sliced apple, a little butter and a pinch of salt.

*Those with a tendency to flatulence should avoid cabbage dishes.

Tender Eggplant

> 1 medium eggplant, washed, peeled and diced
> 1 small onion, chopped

Steam together with a pinch of salt and a pat of butter for 25 minutes. Serve with a cup of broth and a pinch of salt. Garnish with tomato halves or stewed tomatoes.

Steamed or Boiled Vegetable Salads

Carrots, small turnips, beets, beans and cauliflower are especially suited for these salads. Steam the vegetables in water or vegetable stock until tender. Cut into small slices, cubes or strips. Dress with mayonnaise sauce, herb oil dressing or vinaigrette. Use chopped herbs for seasoning.

Potato Salad

> 2 medium potatoes, boiled, peeled and sliced
> 1/2 cup hot vegetable broth.

Pour over potatoes and allow to stand a little while;

Combine and beat together well:

> 1 tablespoon flaxseed or sunflower oil
> 1 tablespoon lemon juice
> 1/2 tablespoon chopped onion
> pinch of salt

Pour dressing mixture over potatoes and let stand a while before serving. Season with parsley, dill, sour milk, mustard or celery seed. You may also enjoy this with 1/4 of a cucumber and some chives grated in.

Rice Salad

Cook 1 cup brown, unpolished rice in
2 cups water. Rinse briefly and allow to cool.

Beat together:
1 tablespoon sunflower oil and
1/2 tablespoon lemon juice

Fold in:
1/2 tablespoon onions and 1/2 tomato, diced fine
Spice with chives, parsley and basil

Mix in with the rice. Serve over lettuce leaves or pastry shells.

Potato Dishes

Potatoes in their Jackets

3 or 4 small potatoes (red or yellow are especially
good), brushed and washed

Place in collander or pan with perforated double-boiler.
Fill pot with water up to the level of the perforated pan, add
a pinch of salt. Put the potatoes inside, cover, and boil 30
or 40 minutes.

Baked Potatoes

2 or 3 potatoes, brushed and washed

Scratch the skin on the upper side of each potato. Paint
each with a little oil and bake 30 to 40 minutes at 350° F
on a greased baking tray. To serve, split each potato open
and lay in a pat of butter.

Parsley Potatoes

2 or 3 potatoes, peeled and quartered, steamed

Melt a tablespoon of butter. Mix in a tablespoon of
chopped parsley and a pinch of salt. Pour over hot potatoes
and serve.

Cottage Cheese Potatoes

2 or 3 potatoes, baked according to above directions

Mix together:

1/2 cup lowfat cottage cheese

1-2 tablespoons milk

chives or caraway seeds

pinch of salt

Stir ingredients together and use as a topping on the hot potatoes.

Caraway Potatoes

2 or 3 medium-large potatoes, washed and cut in half lengthwise.

Mix a teaspoon of bruised caraway seeds with a pinch of salt. Dab the cut surface of the potatoes in the caraway. Place face-down on a greased metal baking sheet. Paint tops with oil and bake 45 minutes at 350° F. For Sesame Potatoes, simply substitute sesame seeds for the caraway.

Bouillon Potatoes

Boil two or three potatoes. In a seperate pan, boil 2 cups vegetable broth, a pinch of salt together with small cubes of leftover carrot, leek, celery or turnips. Boil until vegetables are soft; spread over the potatoes before serving. Season with thyme, bay leaf or parsley.

Mashed potatoes

4 potatoes, peeled, cut up and steamed or boiled until tender, drained

Add a little water or milk to potatoes, then pass through a potato press or process with a masher or food processor.

Add 2 1/2 tablespoons of butter and 1/2 cup milk to

potatoes; stir until foamy. Season with chopped marjoram, caraway, dried tomato, or ground pepper. Serve on a hot dish. Some European cooks like to sculpt the potatoes with a hot, wet knife before serving.

Potato Slices with Spinach

> 1 large potato, peeled and cut lengthwise in quarter-inch slices.

Boil in 2 cups vegetable broth until tender.

Lay them in a single layer on a buttered baking sheet. Take a cup of chopped spinach (recipe above); layer over potatoes. Dot with butter. Season with parsley, chives and nutmeg. Broil dish briefly at 450° F.

Grain or Cereal Dishes

Risotto

> 1/2 cup risotto pasta
> 1/2 cup unpolished rice

Boil together in 2 1/2 cup vegetable broth or water for 30 - 40 minutes.

Mix in a pinch of salt and a pat of butter just before serving; sprinkle with parsley or rosemary.

Tomato Rice

> 1/2 cup unpolished rice
> 1 1/2 cups vegetable broth

Simmer over low heat for 30 to 40 minutes. Add:

> 1 tomato, peeled and cubed.

Mix in a pat of butter and a pinch of salt; season with rosemary, basil or nutmeg.

Rice with Spinach

1 cup spinach, coarsely cut
3/4 cup unpolished rice
3 cups hot vegetable broth

Simmer these together for 30 minutes. Add a pinch of salt and season with basil, peppermint or parsley.

Rice Pudding with Tomatoes

3/4 cup unpolished rice
3 cups vegetable broth
1 tablespoon minced carrots, leeks or celery

Simmer all ingredients together for 30 minutes. Set aside.

Cut three fresh tomatoes into slices.

Layer pudding and tomatoes in a buttered baking pan. Sprinkle with parsley, a little salt and dots of butter. Bake 10 minutes at 325° F.

Sauces

Serve these sauces warm, over rice, pasta or grain dishes

Tomato sauce

2 or 3 tomatoes, cut up and steamed till tender; strained.

Add a little herbal salt and some oregano; a little fresh butter or a tablespoon milk.

Herbal Sauce

Warm 1/2 tablespoon butter. Sprinkle on a tablespoon of flour and stir. Add 1 1/2 cups milk all at once, stir. Add 1/2 cup vegetable broth and simmer 20 minutes. Season with chervil, basil or tarragon.

Vegetable Roast for Special Occasions

This is not a "dietary food" like fresh fruit, vegetables, salads or whole-grain dishes; but they are incomparably more nutritious than meat roasts. When serving, always present a raw vegetable course first; then a soup or salad, and then the "roast" - in this case, an old German recipe. Caraway potatoes are traditionally served with this dish.

Carlsbad Patties
(serves four)
>   2 1/2 cups whole rolled oats, boiled to a thick paste in water or broth

Add:
>   1 large onion, cut into pieces and roasted until yellow

Combine:
>   1 tablespoon butter
>   parsley, celery salt, marjoram and a tablespoon of soy flour.

Mix into oatmeal. Stir well, then grate in:
>   2 or 3 boiled potatoes.

A stiff dough will form. Roll pinches of the dough into 1/4-inch thick patties. Dredge them in whole-wheat flour.

Coat a frying pan with oil, lay in the patties and bake them for 1 hour at 350°F.

Sweet Dishes to Serve 4

Too many sweets and pastries are especially bad for elderly or recovering patients, because sugar promotes fermentation and flatulence. Sugar robs the body of B-vitamins, which are especially important to aging tissues. Instead of commercial white sugar, try using fruit concentrates, honey or fructose.

Berries and Yogurt

Select and wash your choice of strawberries, blueberries, white currants or raspberries: about 1 pint. Mix some fruit concentrate or lemon juice into a pint of plain yogurt, place into single serving bowls or compotes. Decorate the top of the yogurt with the berries.

Fruit Cream

1 pint berries, oranges, or melons, cut up
1 pint lowfat cottage cheese

Mix fruit with lowfat cottage cheese; strain away extra liquid. Add a little lemon juice or fruit concentrate; mix and serve.

Vanilla Cream

2 cups milk
1 vanilla bean, halved lengthwise

Put both into a saucepan and slowly bring milk to a boil.

Stir 2 tablespoons cornstarch together with a little cool milk; stir into the hot pan with a tablespoon of fructose. Bring to a boil again; then allow to cool.

Fruit Salad

Syrup: combine 1 cup of water with 1/4 cup honey; boil. Allow to cool.

Add 1 cup grape juice or other light fruit juice. Set aside.

Combine seasonal fruits to make 4 or 5 cups total: try apricots, peaches, melons, apples, pears, cherries or berries. Cut the fruit into small chunks and put into the syrup. Chill, then serve in small dishes. This is also attractive served in seeded melon halves.

Apple Sauce

> 2 pounds apples, stemmed, peeled, cut up and boiled
> in 2 quarts of water until soft; then strained

Mix in a little fructose, cinnamon and lemon zest. Serve warm or cold. If a smooth apple sauce is desired, whirl the mixture in a blender or food processor before serving.

Blueberry Spread

Good for diarrea sufferers.

> 1 pint blueberries, washed.

Boiled in a quart of water for 5 - 10 minutes. Add a little fructose and a tablespoon of flour, bring to boil. Dot top of mixture with a tablespoon of butter. Pour over toasted bread or bread cubes.

Strawberry Smooth

> 1 cup strawberry slices, washed and trimmed
> 1 1/2 tablespoons fruit concentrate or fructose
> 1 tablespoon lowfat cottage cheese
> 1 tablespoon yogurt

Mix together all ingredients; strain through a sieve. Serve in cups decorated with berry halves. (Don't limit yourself to strawberries: other berries in season work well, too.)

Strawberry or Raspberry Cream

> 1 pint berries
> 1 cup milk
> 1 vanilla bean, split lengthwise

Mix together, strain and bring to a boil together. Serve warm.

Baked Stuffed Apples

4 large or 8 small apples, cored, with grooves cut
   in the skins

Optional filling:

2 tablespoons raisins or currants
1 tablespoon cream
fructose or honey
1 grated lemon peel

Mix together all ingredients, put inside apples and put
together in a baking pan. Drizzle with melted butter; fill each
apple core within 1/4 inch of the top with fruit juice.

Bake at 325°F for 30 minutes. (You may also bake the
apples without the stuffing.)

Lemon-Rice Pudding

Boil together 1 quart water, the juice of one lemon,
diced lemon peel, a pinch of salt, a dribble of honey.

Add 1-1/2 cups of unpolished rice, reduce heat and
simmer, covered for 30 minutes. Remove from heat, allow
to cool. Pour into a jello mold or tube pan; refrigerate.
Serve cold.

Cottage Cheese Pudding

Combine 1/4 cup butter and 4 tablespoons flour in a pan,
brown the flour. Add 1 1/2 cups milk and boil several
minutes.

Mix in a pint of lowfat cottage cheese, 1 beaten egg,
1/4 cup fruit concentrate, 1/2 cup raisins and a grated lemon
peel. Turn into a jello mold or tube pan, bake at 325° F for
30 or 40 minutes. Serve warm.

Health Teas

Chamomile Tea

Infuse a tablespoon of chamomile in a cup of boiling water. Eases stomach pain, cleanses and calms the digestive system. Also used for enemas and douches.

Peppermint Tea

Infuse a tablespoon of peppermint leaves in a cup of boiling water. Calms the stomach and stimulates bile production to speed digestion. This is a popular "pleasure beverage," and makes delicious iced tea.

Rose Hip Tea

Rose hips are available from your health food store; or your neighborhood rose bush. Soak 2 or 3 tablespoons of minced or powdered rose hips and skins in 3 quarts of water for 12 hours. Simmer the liquid slowly for 30 to 45 minutes, then strain. This tea is lightly diuretic (water-shedding) and stimulates digestion. Its lightly-tart flavor makes it a nice compliment to meals.

Linseed Tea

Boil 1 tablespoon of linseeds (flaxseeds) in 2 cups of water for 7 to 10 minutes. It is cleansing and slightly laxative, and helps the body to digest raw fruit juices.

Chapter 7

What Can I Do? Exercise!

It is ironic that prostate sufferers so often find themselves passive recipients of medical treatments. When a disease strikes so close to the "heart" of his manhood, the average man feels he must take an active role in its resolution.

Happily, activity itself can aid in recovery and prevention of prostatitis, prostate hypertrophy and sometimes, prostate cancer. Physicians of cultures throughout the world have developed plans that men themselves work at day-to-day at home, which enables the patient to participate in his own cure.

Men whose problems are not severe can use no-nonsense approaches to improved prostate health. One way is to use the bathroom frequently. "Holding on" simply irritates and stretches the bladder, and can worsen a latent problem.

Going on long car trips can be a trial for a prostate patient, as travel frequently increases the urge to "go." Before leaving on a journey, cut back on caffeine and salty food, which move liquids quickly through the system. As inconvenient as it may be, stop frequently to empty your bladder.

Men who experience *dysuria*, or *"dribbling"* problems, can benefit from *Kegel exercises* - an internal workout that strengthens the muscles in the lower pelvis. Popularized by proponents of Natural Childbirth and named for the doctor who discovered its benefits, this squeezing motion can help men with weak urine streams better control their bladder muscles.

INSTRUCTIONS
Kegel Exercise

To do a Kegel exercise, simply squeeze the muscles you'd normally use to hold back or stop a stream of urine. Hold for a count of three, then release for a count of three. Repeat 25 times, three times a day. The "workout" is perfectly silent and still, and can be done in the midst of a day's work without notice or undue exertion.

Along with a change in diet, *exercise* is the easiest, least expensive habit a man can develop to *keep his prostate healthy*.

Exercise doesn't necessarily mean strenuous weight-lifting or long hours of racquet-swinging. The one form of exercise that is far superior to any other for prostate maintenance is *walking*.

The splendid aspect of *walking* is its simplicity. No fancy, expensive equipment is needed; there's no need to visit a personal trainer for "walking lessons." Anyone who is not handicapped can walk. It promotes togetherness and conversation, making it an ideal workout for couples. Regular evening walks may even put some romance back into your life!

If prostate health - and perhaps your future sexual health - aren't impetus enough to get you off the sofa and walking around the block, perhaps these facts will help.

Daily walking, even as little as 30 minutes, has these effects on the human body:

1. It lowers your chances of having a heart attack.

In a continuing study of Harvard University alumni, researchers find that men who burn at least 2,000 calories a week walking or doing other moderate exercise have a 28 percent lower death rate from cardiac problems than those who do little or no exercise. This and other studies show that a regular walking program lowers a man's blood pressure and his resting heart rate.

2. It lowers levels of artery-clogging blood fats.

This works hand-in-hand with a lowered risk of heart attack, but also benefits the arteries that supply blood to the genitals and enable a man to get an erection. Men whose arteries are clogged with cholesterol fats may not have sufficient blood flow to create a firm erection.

Walking lowers these blood fats that narrow arteries and increases levels of HDL, the "good cholesterol" that fights fatty buildup.

3. It controls body weight.

Walking increases your body's metabolism, which burns calories. Exercise increases the conversion of fat cells to energy, and builds muscle tissue, which in turn burns more calories. Regular walking also tends to curb your appetite.

4. It improves mental outlook.

A good workout releases *endorphins*, natural mood-elevating brain chemicals. Walking can actually put you in a good mood. A recent study showed that walking is more effective than tranquilizers at relieving anxiety.

5. It relieves back pain.

Walking strengthens and tones muscles that stabilize the spine. Unlike jogging, walking puts little stress on the spinal disks and knee and ankle joints. In fact, walking puts less stress on your spine than sitting does!

6. It increases energy.

Instead of eating a candy bar when you need a quick burst of energy, try taking a 10-minute walk. Dr. Robert Thayer, a professor at California State University, headed a study that found a walk as short as 10 minutes not only produces extra energy, but a burst that outlasts the "power boost" of a candy bar. Walkers also display less muscle tension than their candy-munching counterparts, Thayer found.

Chuck N. says he's a living example of the benefits of walking. When he was a young man, Chuck didn't have a car. He walked to work, to dates, to the store and back, never thinking twice about "exercise." He had little choice.

As he grew older, Chuck continued to walk —now to work and appointments. By then he had a car of his own, but used it only for longer trips.

Today, Chuck is a strapping, healthy 95-year-old. He's never had a problem with his prostate, he says, and continues to walk every day.

Massage and Prostate Problems

One of the best ways to soothe an irritated prostate is to massage it. Many urologists bring patients needed relief by stroking the gland with a gloved finger. The doctor accesses the gland anally, then presses down on the prostate, beginning at the top and working toward the bottom. This empties the gland of excess secretions and reduces its size enough to provide temporary relief. It works by stimulating circulation to the gland, which in turn reduces inflammation.

Many doctors advise patients like Howard H. to massage their own prostate glands. Howard visited his doctor because he couldn't urinate - his prostate had swollen to twice its normal size. His hips ached, and a intermittent fever sometimes reached 101 degrees F.

The doctor massaged Howard's prostate, then advised him to buy some rubber finger cots at the drugstore. Finger cots are rubber tubes that fit snugly over a finger. With this equipment, Howard continued his treatment at home. (Some men prefer to use less-expensive condoms, some of which are manufactured with a lubricant.)

INSTRUCTIONS
Prostate Massage

Consult your doctor before beginning this procedure: improper massage may further irritate your prostate.

This is best done in a sitting position, usually on a toilet seat or standing, with one foot on a chair.

Cover index finger with a cot. Insert the finger about 1 1/2 inch into rectum. Very gently stroke the rounded shape of the prostate just as your doctor does, starting at the top and working toward the bottom. The massage may be done every other day, or even daily, depending on your condition and doctor's advice.

Reflexology

Reflexology is a system of physical culture that is based on therapeutic massage. By massaging various reflex points of the body, you not only eliminate pain in the region being massaged, but also release healing energy throughout the body.

You may be familiar with these reflex points if you've heard of acupuncture. Practitioners of this ancient Chinese healing method teach that these points are energy junctions that relay and reinforce energy along the body's "meridian lines," which send vital energy through the organs via the nervous system.

Reflexologists don't use needles, however. They use their hands and fingers to massage the reflex points, releasing endorphins into the body tissues. These "feel-good" neurotransmitters suppress pain and produce a calming or even euphoric effect on the body. It's the same chemical that produces the long-distance "runner's high."

Reflexologist Mildred Carter, author of the book *Body Reflexology: Healing At Your Fingertips*, writes that men can use this massage system to alleviate prostate symptoms. Dale L., 22, avoided prostate surgery by using reflexology.

After Dale's BPH diagnosis, he visited several doctors and specialists, seeking a non-surgical answer to his dilemma. They all recommended prostate surgery, but Dale felt he was too young for that.

After reading up on *reflexology*, Dale began stimulating the "reflex buttons" on his wrists (see diagram).

After only two weeks of regular massage, Dale's prostate problems were gone, including a bad case of nocturia - the need to urinate frequently at night. He wrote: "I feel like

I should have been feeling all these years - energetic - and I have a new lease on life. I feel better now than I can ever remember feeling all my life."

Massaging Reflexes of the Hand

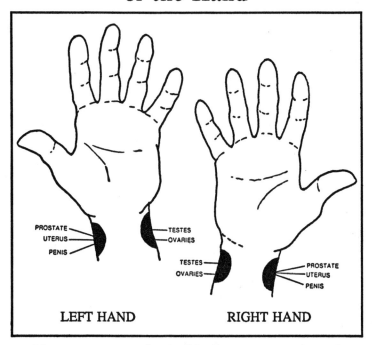

LEFT HAND   RIGHT HAND

Nerve centers associated with the prostate are located directly beneath the thumbs, about an inch below the wrist.

To make use of this Oriental cure, simply massage the same area on both wrists several times a day. If there is tenderness or pain, continue to gently massage. This indicates a problem with the organ or gland being treated, Carter says.

Other prostate-related reflex buttons are located on the feet, on the outside, below and slightly behind the protrusion of the ankle bone. Massage here will also bring prostate relief.

Massaging Reflexes of the Foot

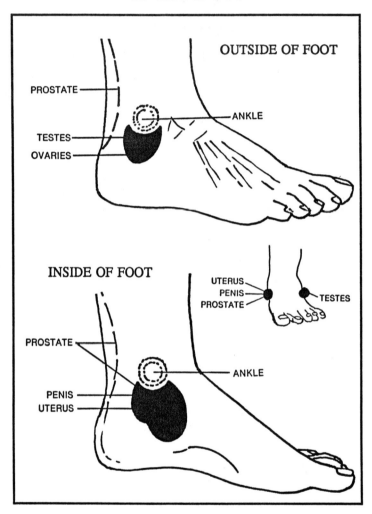

If neither of these points works for you after two weeks of massage, get to the root of the problem. Massage the area around the base of the penis with your fingertips. If this band of muscle feels hard to the touch, massage it until the hardness vanishes and the tissue is pliable, Carter advises.

Internal Exercises: Move Your Chi Around

Over 2,500 years ago, the Chinese developed *Tao*, (rhymes with "plow") a philosophy of serenity and longevity for mind, body, spirit and society. "Chi" is a word for the body's natural healing energy. Integral to Tao - and Buddhism - is a system of fitness called "Tai Chi." Its elegant, dancelike movements are frequently portrayed in documentaries and martial arts demonstrations. I don't intend to teach Tai Chi, but only touch on an unseen aspect of its discipline: the internal exercise.

Dr. Stephen T. Chang, author of *The Complete System of Self-Healing: Internal Exercises*, writes of the benefits of putting the body's natural healing energy to work on specific internal organs and glands.

For clarity's sake I will explain a basic philosophy shared by Tao, Zen, Hinduism and other Eastern religions - the existence of several nerve centers, what the Indians call *chakras*, laid in a pathway "from top to tail." When the body is healthy, energy can travel freely from one *chakra* to another, finally reaching the pineal gland, or "head chakra," the seat of spirituality.

When practiced regularly, internal exercises balance the body's energy level and promote more effective functions in major organs. Thus is the body better able to heal its injuries, adjust to environmental changes, correct abnormalities and fight disease.

Internal exercises can help your body heal prostatic problems and improve your spirituality and sex life, too, Tao experts assert. The best prostate exercise is called the *Deer Exercise*. It is said to not only prevent, but also reverse *prostatitis* and *prostatic hypertrophy*.

Contemplating nature is an important element of Tao practice, and the sages who developed the internal exercises reflect this contemplation in the names they give the practices. Three long-lived animals: the deer, turtle and crane, inspired series of exercises the sages derived from observing them.

The deer was admired for his strong sexual and reproductive powers. The wise men noticed that dominant stags exercised their anal muscles every time they twitched their tails, and an exercise was born.

INSTRUCTIONS
Deer Exercise

Stage One: Rub the palms of your hands together to bring your body's energy to your hands.

Place the palm of your right hand over your testicles, completely covering them but not squeezing.

Place the palm of your left hand on your pubic bone - about an inch below your navel. Move your left hand slowly in a clockwise circle 81 times, exerting only slight pressure on the pubis.

Rub your palms together again.

Reverse the position of your hands, placing your left hand over your testicles and your right hand on your pubis - the bony ridge at the base of your belly. Repeat the 81 circles, but in a counter-clockwise direction.

Concentrate on the energy moving between your two palms. This is extremely important, Chang asserts, as it unifies body and mind. *Continued...*

Deer Exercises, *continued*

If you get an erection during the exercise, take the hand from your testicles and place it over the base of your penis. Press down sharply while massaging the pubis area with the other hand. This inhibits blood flow to the penis and maximizes energy build-up within your internal sex glands.

Stage Two: Stand with hands in the Stage One position. Tighten the muscles of your anus, drawing them upward and inward. It should feel as if air is being drawn into your rectum. Tighten as much as possible and hold this position as long as it is comfortable.

Stop and rest for a moment, then repeat the anal contraction as many times as is comfortable. (If this reminds you of the Kegel Exercise explained above, you are correct - it works out the same muscle group.)

While you squeeze, concentrate on the sensations traveling along the pathway between your belly, back, throat and head - the chi flowing along your internal pathway. Don't force this sensation with mental images. It will occur naturally, and last for only a fraction of a second.

At first, it may be difficult to hold the contraction for longer than a few seconds. After several weeks, though, there should be a noticeable improvement. To test the effectiveness of the *Deer Exercise,* try to stop your urine stream when you use the bathroom through use of anal contractions. If you can stop the flow - say thank-you to the Tao Masters!

During the *Deer Exercise,* the tightening anal muscles gently massage the prostate gland. The gland in turn secretes endorphins, those friendly "feel-good" chemicals. Other advantages include increased sensitivity around the pubis and penis, which may help with impotence and premature ejaculation. Moreover, the Tao Masters believed the *Deer Exercise* enlarges the bulb at the penis' tip, which gives a man more pleasurable intercourse.

For maximum benefit, do the *Deer Exercise* twice each day, morning and night.

Another simple Chinese exercise designed to increase circulation to the sex glands is described below.

INSTRUCTIONS
Sexual Glands Exercise

Sit on the floor and bend your knees so that the soles of your feet touch in front of your body.

Rub the bottoms of your feet together until they are warm - then put them together.

Rub your toes with your fingers until they are warm.

With your feet held together, draw your heels up toward your pelvis as close as is comfortable. Hold your toes with your hands, and, using your elbows, press your knees toward the floor.

Rub the insides of your thighs with your palms. Start at the knees and continue massaging upward to the inner pelvis. Repeat this massage seven times.

Gently pummel your inner thighs with your fists to stimulate blood circulation and energy in your legs and sexual organs. Continue the exercise as long as comfort allows.

Answers from India

Yoga is another program brought to us from far away in space and time. Physicians are now accepting this 5,000-year-old Indian therapy for the curative physical therapy program it is.

According to doctors at the Yoga Research Laboratory at Lonavla, India, one simple Yoga "pose" is especially beneficial to prostate sufferers: it is called the *Kneeling Pose*. *The Yoga Mudra* requires a bit more flexibility. It increases circulation to the genital area. It also works the colon muscles and relieves constipation - but don't try these exercises on a full stomach, or if you have arthritis or other problems with your joints.

INSTRUCTIONS
Yoga Kneeling Pose

Sit on your heels on the floor, your back straight. Relax. SLOWLY separate your feet and let your bottom sink between until it touches the floor. Repeat 15 times or more, being careful not to twist your knee joints.

Yoga Mudra Pose

Sit cross-legged on the floor. Let out your breath, and slowly lean forward until your forehead touches the floor in front of you. Reach behind your back and grasp the wrist of one hand in the other. Hold for a count of five, inhale, and slowly rise back to a sitting position. Repeat up to 15 minutes.

More Sex

Other suggested therapies are practiced worldwide: the most popular is espoused by Stephen N. Rous, M.D., author of *The Prostate Book*. His suggested cure for nonbacterial prostate problems is more sex.

Rous reasons that a decrease in sexual release can cause ejaculate to accumulate in the prostate to the point of pain. Indeed, many men - especially younger ones - complain of this mysterious "blue balls" ailment when their partners cannot or will not cooperate with their sexual wishes.

More sex is a favorite therapy for many when prostate symptoms flare up - I won't include instructions for it here! But be sure to discuss with your doctor any symptom that returns regularly or impedes sexual performance.

Baths: Circulizer and Sitzbath

For almost 40 years, Europeans have treated circulatory and vascular problems with a method that makes use of "consensual reaction" theory, also known as the *Dastre-Moratsche* reaction.

This reaction is illustrated best by the old adage: "Get cold feet, get a cold." A second look at Mom's warnings about getting your feet wet on a chilly day may hold scientific water: a shock to the cold receptors in the feet can effectively lower temperatures in a patient's mouth, sinuses and outer ear canals - which may just make him more susceptible to catching a cold.

Doctors Dastre and Moratsche put a reverse spin on these findings, and came up with a warming footbath therapy that gets good results on thousands of European users.

Their bath unit, marketed as the *F-S Circulizer* in the United States, uses a slowly rising temperature and several healing herbs to expand the tiny capillaries in the soles of the feet. As the water temperature rises, the blood vessels in the feet expand to maximum, starting a chain reaction of dilation throughout the circulatory system.

Extensive testing has shown the circulizer effective in dealing with *impotency, colds, flu, bronchitis, angina, bladder irregularities, asthma, migraine headaches, dizziness, insomnia, arthritis, prostate problems, osteoporosis, low and high blood pressure, varicose veins, lupus* and many more ailments.

This method is especially helpful for men whose prostates aren't the only organ with problems, and whose medical conditions preclude surgery.

One 83-year-old subject had a heart condition. His advanced age, coupled with the cardiac problem and a prostate the size of a chicken egg made him turn to the circulizer as a last resort. Even the weakest heart isn't endangered by a foot bath, so his doctor consented.

Four weeks later, the same doctor expressed amazement at his patient's marked improvement. The elderly man's prostate had returned to normal size.

Sitz Baths

Many doctors recommend prostate patients take hot *sitzbaths* to shrink their swollen glands. Naturopathic doctor Paavo Airola frequently prescribed them to his patients.

The water should be as hot as you can stand. About 8 inches of water usually is enough; you should sit in the bath with knees drawn up toward your chest. Stay in the water for 10 to 15 minutes; repeat two or three times a week. In most cases, the hot water alone provides relief from inflammation. But those with acute problems may want to add some *chamomile tea* to the bath.

INSTRUCTIONS
Chamomile Tea

Preparation: Boil one pint of water and add one ounce of chamomile blossoms. Cover the pot tightly and steep for 10 to 12 minutes; don't let vapor escape with the medicinal qualities.

Strain out the leaves, pour the liquid into the hot bath water.

Specialized Exercise Program for Men

Many natural health adherents have discovered a low-impact exercise method that is proven to improve cardiopulmonary fitness and condition the body systems that serve the prostate gland.

This device was used by former President Ronald Reagan during his White House years, when he couldn't get outdoors to exercise. Studies by NASA and the US Air Force found the rebounder exerciser 68 percent more effective than jogging, providing measurable reductions in body fat and high improvement in fitness levels.

The Rebounder is an exercise apparatus now in use by former U.S. National Champion weightlifter John Orsini. The hefty athlete describes it as the "ultimate stress-free way to work out, especially for men who want to start a fitness program but need to start out slowly."

Rebounding:
The Exercise of Choice

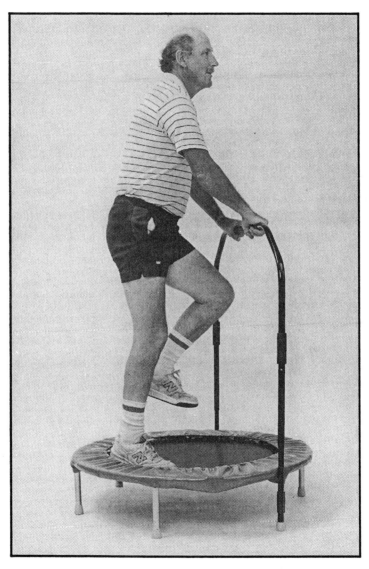

No matter what your age, the Airo-Bounder helps you
regain youthful vitality.

Rebounding exercisers trace their origins to the trampoline, a bouncy platform invented in 1936 and used extensively by athletes and trainers through the World War II era to develop coordination, timing and flexibility. Pole vaulters, gymnasts, wrestlers, soccer players and skiers still make good use of trampolines in their training programs.

Trampolines became popular in schools and fitness facilities during the 1950s and '60s - kids enjoyed the high flying and bouncing so much they didn't realize how much exercise they were getting. Unfortunately, a lack of supervision and abuse by daredevils gave the trampoline an early exit from public schools.

The first modern *rebounders* appeared in the 1970s; they were little more than mini-trampolines. These apparatus developed through time; sturdy handrails, stiffer springs and a more even tension were added. The "mini-tramp" became an effective training machine.

Rebounding has become the exercise of choice for many Americans who previously hesitated to jump into the fitness craze. A jogging or walking motion on a rebounder provides all the exercise of normal motion without the steady pounding experienced by runners, joggers and walkers, making it an ideal exerciser for diabetics and those recovering from injuries or surgery. The firm "bounce-back" of the polypropylene mat builds endurance levels and lower-body muscles, but pampers joints and tendons.

Many folks new to exercise are shy about working out in a gym or health club. Others don't have more than a few minutes each day to give to exercise, or can't leave home or office for the time it takes to work out.

Rebounding is the ideal answer to all these dilemmas. No special wardrobe, membership fee, transportation or time demands are required - you can "bound" in the privacy of your home, whatever the weather, in your undershorts if you like! And the unit folds easily into a carrying case for easy storage and travel.

And the bottom line is less than $200: much "healthier" on the pocketbook than many other exercisers on the market!

The Physical Specifications of the Airo-Bounder ™

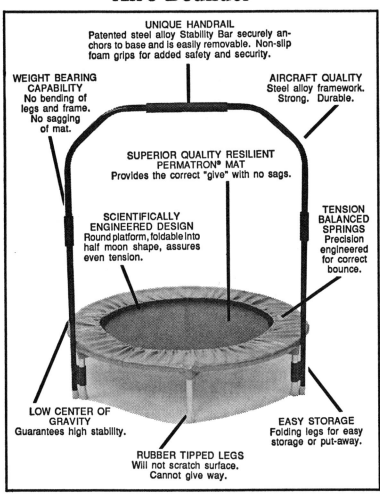

UNIQUE HANDRAIL
Patented steel alloy Stability Bar securely anchors to base and is easily removable. Non-slip foam grips for added safety and security.

WEIGHT BEARING CAPABILITY
No bending of legs and frame. No sagging of mat.

AIRCRAFT QUALITY
Steel alloy framework. Strong. Durable.

SUPERIOR QUALITY RESILIENT PERMATRON® MAT
Provides the correct "give" with no sags.

SCIENTIFICALLY ENGINEERED DESIGN
Round platform, foldable into half moon shape, assures even tension.

TENSION BALANCED SPRINGS
Precision engineered for correct bounce.

LOW CENTER OF GRAVITY
Guarantees high stability.

EASY STORAGE
Folding legs for easy storage or put-away.

RUBBER TIPPED LEGS
Will not scratch surface. Cannot give way.

Dr. James R. White wrote that rebounding for a sufficient amount of time each week changes and improves every cell in the body, increasing endurance, aerobic capacity and cardiovascular health.

The key to rebounding is gravity; putting nature's resistance to work for you. Bouncing isn't necessary. Even those recovering from serious illness can put the bounder to good use by sitting on the platform, grasping the stability bar and pulling their body upward by their arms.

Testimonial letters on file at the Rebound Fitness Society attest to the program's effectiveness:

"I'm in my 80's, and exercise was the farthest thing from my mind," wrote C.S. of Menlo Park, CA. *"My son gave me a rebounder and set it up for me. I tried it only because I felt obligated to him.*

"It amazed me. It was delightful. And I really have noticed a substantial improvement in my stamina. My balance seems better; I no longer have that "tottery" feeling. I'm not troubled as much by arthritis. It's really given me a new lease on life. No more rocking chair for me!"

The Rebound Fitness Society has exercise programs for overweight, aged, athletes and average people alike. Those interested in more information on this unique exercise program may contact:

The Rebound Fitness Society
P.O. Box 116, Dept. A
Canfield, OH 44406
(216) 533-5673

Chapter 8

Prostate Cancer
The Big C and
"Establishment"
Treatments

Prostate cancer is a disease most men know little about - and would rather not think on. But like it or not, prostate cancer awareness is growing.

A prostate cancer screening booth was set up at the 1992 Republican National Convention, at the urging of Senatorial prostate patient Bob Dole. 1993's rash of celebrity deaths from prostate cancer - actors Telly Savalas, Don Ameche and Bill Bixby, musician Frank Zappa and entertainment mogul Steve Ross - served to launch the "quiet killer" into the feature pages of *Newsweek* and *Time* and into the national consciousness.

Prostate cancer strikes one man in eight. But it is a slow-growing type of cancer, and usually occurs in men over 60. Most males don't take the danger seriously, doctors say.

Anything having to do with elimination or reproduction causes squeamishness in many Americans - most of whom are also taught to "be a man" and "tough it out" when faced with pain or illness.

When they first consider the standard medical options, it's no wonder so many newly diagnosed men retreat into denial. The prostate's complicated location, amidst a tangle of nerve bundles and muscle groups, makes it notoriously difficult to operate on or treat with radiation without damaging surrounding tissue. Resulting impotence and incontinence may be "a fate worse than death" to some men.

As medical ethicist Arthur Caplan told *Newsweek*: "There isn't a right answer (to prostate cancer patients.) You can choose to have the surgery, if what matters to you is long life and you don't care if you become impotent or have a harder time peeing. Or someone at age 70 might decide, 'I'm not buying enough time to put those functions at risk'."

Early prostate cancer symptoms are identical to those of BPH and prostatitis, so most doctors will run routine blood and urine tests on any prostate patient to ensure that cancer cells aren't present. A debate is raging over how widespread early detection tests should become, and who should pay for them. But instead of arguing public policy, I will discuss the disease itself.

What is Prostate Cancer?

Experts haven't yet discovered what causes prostate cancer, but they have connected it to high levels of the hormones testosterone and estradiol. They suspect that high-fat diets may stimulate production of these hormones.

Other links have been found in patients' heredity, sexual

practices, past history of illness, injury or surgery. (One study found that men who'd undergone vasectomies sometimes had a higher incidence of prostate cancer later on.)

Cancer is, basically, the body's own cells gone awry. When normal cells' growth processes are effected over time by *carcinogens* - cancer-causing agents - they sometimes "mutate" into cancer cells. These maverick cells grow more rapidly than usual, and "take over" neighboring cells' growth apparatus. A cancer that starts in a particular organ frequently changes the blood chemistry or secretions of the organ, giving doctors a chemical warning sign.

In 1992, 35,000 men died after cancer cells in their prostates migrated — or *metastasized* — to their bones.

More than 80 percent of these men were age 60 or over. About 60 percent of them were diagnosed while the cancer was still localized in their prostate glands. 88 percent of them lived at least five years beyond their diagnosis. Prostate cancer kills if not treated on time. Early detection is therefore of great importance.

These numbers place prostate cancer as the second-most deadly cancer among American men, just behind lung cancer. Healthcare experts estimate that if all 20 million at-risk American men were tested for prostate cancer, 400,000 would be found eligible for treatment. For now, about 100,000 new cases are diagnosed each year.

Prostate cancer usually grows very slowly, and frequently stays right where it is instead of spreading through the body. Many men have prostate cancer for years and never know it - many cancers are found only after BPH treatments provide sample tissues. Postmortem exams frequently find undiagnosed prostate cancer in bodies that expired from an unrelated illness.

But in other instances, doctors do find cancer, usually through a rectal exam. This 10-minute procedure is recommended by the American Cancer Society, which says every man over 40 should include one in his annual checkup. Doctors sometimes use an instrument called a *sigmoidoscope* to view the interior of the colon, where they look for internal cysts, hemorrhoids or abnormal tissue.

Others settle for the rubber glove approach; many men find a *digital examination* more comfortable, if not as comprehensive.

Digital Examination for Prostate Cancer

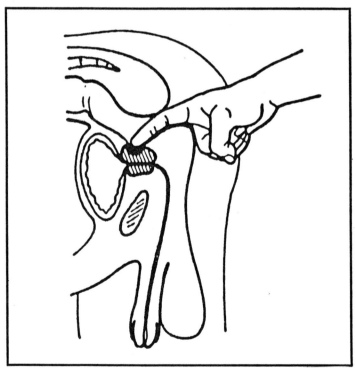

Pschyrembel Klinisches Wörterbuch. DeGruyter, Berlin, Germany. 1986.

Those at risk for cancer can undergo a blood test that detects abnormal amounts of *prostatic specific antigen (PSA)*, a cancer indicator. (Critics say this test is usually accurate only about 60 percent of the time, however.) Dr. Isadore Rosenfeld describes these tests in his recent book *The Best Treatment*, and writes that abnormally high PSA readings usually prompt an *acid phosphatase test*, which tells if prostate cancer has metastasized to the bones.

Other routine diagnostic tools include *fine needle aspiration* or *needle biopsy* - removal of a bit of the prostate tissue through an anally-administered needle.

Prostatic Aspiration
To Determine the Presence or
Absence of Prostatic Cancer

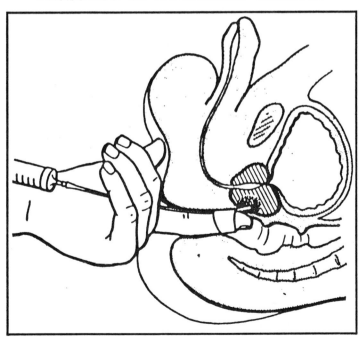

Pschyrembel Klinisches Wörterbuch. DeGruyter, Berlin, Germany. 1986.

If a final diagnosis isn't obtained through this outpatient procedure, the doctor may schedule an ultrasound-guided laparascopic exam, similar to the TURP apparatus used to surgically reduce prostatic hypertrophy. (Rosenfeld calls this a "biopsy gun.") This secures bits of prostate tissue that should secure a diagnosis, and can sometimes be done in a urologist's office.

If the diagnosis is cancer, several options can be considered. If the cancer is still limited to the prostate gland, there are several choices, each with its avid advocates.

1. Watchful Waiting. This is the best option for those who are elderly, uninsured, in poor health or have cancer samples that are "well-differentiated," or somewhat stable. Your doctor will want you to return to his office every three or four months for rectal exams and PSA tests. If and when the cancer begins to spread, more aggressive action can be taken. Those opposed to this approach, like *Newsweek* magazine health writer Jerry Adler, say this "amounts to monitoring the tumor in expectation that something else will kill the patient first."

2. Radiation is another cancer treatment option with its share of advocates and nay-sayers. Dr. Rosenfeld writes that his patients find their long-term outlook is better with radiation than "watchful waiting;" as many as 85 percent live at least 10 more years. "Seeding" a tumor with radioactive pellets the size of a rice grains is a popular treatment. It is less invasive and expensive than surgery, but it requires expert handling. Troublesome side effects include chronic diarrhea, exhaustion, rectal pain and fissures, incontinence, infections and impotence.

3. Radical Prostatectomy, or surgical removal of the prostate, either through an abdominal incision gives about the same chance for cure as radiation. It is the treatment of choice of American urologists: a 1988 survey said 80 percent of these doctors would recommend the surgery to a man in his 60s whose cancer was confined to the gland. In England, however, only 4 percent of the urologists said they would recommend the surgery; 92 percent of American radiation oncologists said they would advise against it.

Prostatectomy is a serious abdominal operation. It is risky, expensive, and of questionable value to men over 70 years old, according to a recent Dartmouth University study. Eight percent of men studied over age 75 suffered serious complications after the surgery; 2 percent died of them.

Radical Prostatectomy leaves up to 85 percent of patients impotent; 27 percent of patients are at least partially incontinent. New "nerve-sparing" surgical techniques are improving the odds for men concerned about sexual vigor, however; and researchers say that less invasive surgical techniques are in the works.

The Dartmouth team told *Newsweek* that "if the medical community were to apply the same standards of safety and efficacy required for approval of new drugs... it is likely that neither *radical prostatectomy* nor *radiation therapy* would be approved."

Even though thousands of men are treated with surgeries that have few scientific studies to back them, the news is not all bad. Just look at Bob Dole, 71, Republican leader of the US Senate. His prostate was removed in 1991, but his aggressive energy is the bane of Democrats everywhere.

Cryosurgery is the newest wave in prostate cancer surgery. With the patient under general anaesthesia, doctors insert five metal probes between the scrotum and anus, eliminating the need for a deep incision. After placing the probes about the prostate with help from ultrasound imaging, the doctor then injects super-cooled nitrogen into the cancerous tissues. A computer monitors tissue destruction through the ultrasound system. The procedure requires only one night in the hospital, and causes little or no bleeding. Recovery is quick, and sexual potency is frequently spared.

Laser Surgery is still experimental in *prostate cancer* cases, but some doctors see it as the surgery of choice for the future. Currently it is used as an alternative to TURP or *radical prostatectomy*, as a way to eliminate the cancerous gland altogether without opening the abdomen. Laser surgery is easy on the patient. It causes no bleeding or long recovery time, can be used with little or no anesthetic, can be repeated without ill effects and is virtually painless.

Testosterone, a male hormone produced in the testicles, effectively "feeds" prostate cancer, researchers have found. Many men have the problem removed at its source, by having their testes surgically removed in an operation known as "orchiectomy." It is the oldest form of hormone treatment for *prostate cancer*, and is frequently used to treat *testicular cancer*, as well.

Rosenfeld recommends this surgical castration, even though he admits it sounds brutal. The operation can be done in a day, and small plastic balls are inserted into the scrotal sac for appearance's sake. This inevitably ends in impotence, however.

Non-Surgical Options

Hormone therapies are as popular as surgeries, but are dismissed by many urologists as unproven. Many patients whose cancer has metastasized find relief through reducing the amount of male hormone in the bloodstream - the substance the cancer "feeds on." Without testosterone, impotency is almost inevitable.

One such drug is *diethylstibestrol (DES)*, a chemical similar to estrogen, a female hormone. Although DES brings with it a longer life and lessened symptoms, it isn't without side effects. It kills a man's sex drive, and many men report feminizing effects: breast enlargement, thinning beards and scrotal shrinkage.

LH-RH Agonists (Leuprolide and *Goserelin)* can be used to treat even later stages of prostate cancer. This synthetic pituitary hormone therapy regulates the release of testosterone into the blood stream. After triggering an initial rush of *testosterone*, it causes a drastic decrease in *testosterone*, which "starves" the tumor. Its only remarkable side effect is occasional hot flashes, headaches or impotence. The agonists are usually administered through injections or implanted pellets.

LH-RH's inevitable downside is its longevity - effectiveness sometimes decreases after two years. It also effects only the pituitary gland, not the testosterone-producing cells in the testes. The small amount produced "down there" may be enough to keep a stray cancer cell or two alive.

Antiandrogens are hormones that inhibit the action of testosterone on cancer cells. Marketed through the brand name *Flutamide*, antiandrogens are frequently used in concord with other hormone treatments to lessen the pain of advanced prostate cancer.

Dr. Fernand LaBrie, a physician of the Department of Molecular Endocrinology at Laval University Medical Center in Quebec, uses a "one-two punch" on his prostate cancer patients. He combines a *Luprolide-type drug* with Flutamide, and reports a 70 percent response rate to this therapy.

The Prostate Gland Showing the Different Stages of Cancer

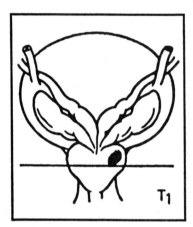

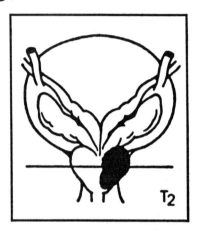

STAGE T1 - Cancer is palpable on digital examination. It is small in size and is localized to one side of the prostate gland.

STAGE T2 - A more extensive form of cancer infiltration — detected through digital examination. Where it is thought that the cancer has not spread outside of the prostate gland.

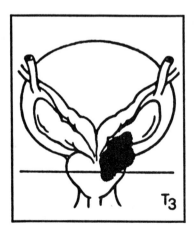

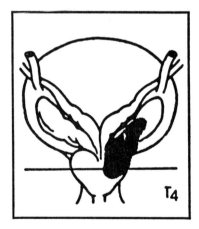

STAGE T3 - Cancer is one in which the prostate cancer has spread outside the confines of the prostate gland. Detectable through digital examination.

STAGE T4 - Cancer has spread outside the confines of the prostate gland and has metastasized.

Immunotherapy is a method used to build up the body's natural defenses against all diseases, including cancer. Some doctors combine *immunotherapy* with *chemotherapy* to help patients through later stages of prostate cancer. Other sufferers use natural cures and herbal soothers to help their bodies fight the cancer. Some of these are detailed in chapter 9.

Medical Investigational Treatments

Some doctors are seeing successful results from several new prostate cancer treatments - used alone or in combination with other treatment options. Be aware that these methods are used only on an experimental basis, and it can take up to 15 years for scientists to prove the long-term effectiveness of any experimental option. Your doctor can inform you on where and what clinical trials are ongoing in your region. Ask him to contact the National Cancer Institute's Physicians' Direct Query, or "PDQ" referral system.

Radiation and "Hyperthermia"

Scientists know that temperatures of 106 degrees Fahrenheit or above are deadly to cell division and weak cells. They are attempting to put this information to work on prostate cancer by combining it with radiation to kill cancer cells.

Dr. Isaac Kaver of the University of Virginia wrote in the medical journal *Urology* that heat makes cancer cells more sensitive to radiation. Application of heat to the whole body or to the localized tumor area and then to radiation was more effective at killing the cells than using either treatment alone, Kaver wrote.

High Energy Radiation

Another variation on standard radiation therapy is *high linear energy transfer radiation*. Instead of using the usual X-ray or gamma ray radiation, this method employs "accelerators" that use helium ions, neutrons and protons to penetrate to deep-seated tumors and irradiate the cancer tissues. Some experts say this is more effective than standard radiation therapy. Its is available, however, at only a few sites throughout the continent.

Enzyme-Inhibiting Drugs are already in use for treatment of benign prostatic hypertrophy. *Finasteride (Proscar)*, a new drug discussed in chapter 3, is also being studied as an early-stage cancer treatment. *Finasteride* works by blocking production of an enzyme that triggers production of a testosterone by-product that "feeds" prostate tumors. *Suramin*, a drug with exotic origins, is also being studied. Originally used to treat African Sleeping Sickness, some researchers are finding it interferes with tumor growth.

Chemotherapy is usually considered a last resort for cancer patients. It uses chemicals to directly attack cancer cells, but usually ends up killing many healthy cells as well. However, an experimental group of 25 men written up in Urology showed a significant (50 percent) drop in PSA levels after being treated with a combination of standard chemotherapy drugs.

Biological Therapy

Like the immunotherapy option listed above, this experimental method involves use of substances meant to trigger the body's natural defenses against disease.

Colony-stimulating factors are produced within the body and trigger production of white blood cells - the body's disease-defenders. Scientists say use of colony-stimulators allows higher doses of chemotherapy to be used to target the cancer directly.

T-Cells recognize and attack cancer cells. Scientists are experimenting with removing *T-cells* from the blood, fortifying them and boosting their reproduction, then returning them to the body to attack the cancer. *Tumor necrosis factors* are tumor-destroying proteins. Scientists are trying to find a way to trigger increased production of these proteins within the body.

Other researchers are working on "designer proteins" called *monoclonal antibodies*. These natural cancer-attackers go after specific types of cancer. Doctors hope to someday attach medication or radiation to these proteins to better deliver relief to the affected organs and tissues.

The Mayo Clinic Health Letter recently reported on another experiment with proteins called *interleukins* and *interferons* - substances the body makes to fight off infections. Scientists hope to synthesize these proteins for injection into cancer patients.

All of these therapies are still being worked out on the cellular level, under the microscopes of scientists throughout the world. Although they hold hope for future cancer patients, the man recently diagnosed may be hard-pressed to find a local doctor who is well-informed on every aspect of current research.

Oncogene Therapy is a genetic approach to cancer treatment. Scientists recently discovered that normal genes - the tiny protein chains that carry a cell's genetic information - can sometimes, somehow, change into cancer-promoting genes called *oncogenes*.

An upbeat accompaniment was discovery of *suppressor genes* - a concurrent group of genes that sometimes forestall production of oncogenes. As detailed in Shapiro's *Prostate Problems* book, the discovery opens up a new realm of treatment possibilities - *"gene therapy"* for cancer-prone patients. Doctors may someday replace oncogenes or faulty suppressor genes with "good" genes.

Metastasis: Stopping the Spread

Scientists at the National Cancer Institute have recently found several new clues as to why cancer spreads, and are working on therapies that could stop cancer where it starts. A piece in *The Scientific American* detailed the breakthroughs.

Metalloproteinases, enzymes secreted by cancer cells, were linked to metastasis by several researchers. They are working on ways to inhibit production or change the composition of these enzymes, which break down the defensive cell walls of healthy tissues and allow cancer cells to invade.

Caring for your Testicles

Another threat men face from "down there" is *orchitis*, or *inflammation of the testes*, and *cancer of the testes*.

Orchitis can strike younger men as well as the middle-aged and elderly, and it is frequently "let go to pass on its own" by men too embarrassed to consult with a doctor. Unfortunately, overlooking a case of *orchitis* could result in later infertility.

Orchitis, like *prostatitis*, is frequently caused by a bacterial infection inside the organs - not necessarily venereal disease. *Orchitis* can indicate *tuberculosis* or *mumps infections* elsewhere in the body.

Crossection of Male Genitourinary Tract
(DETAIL)

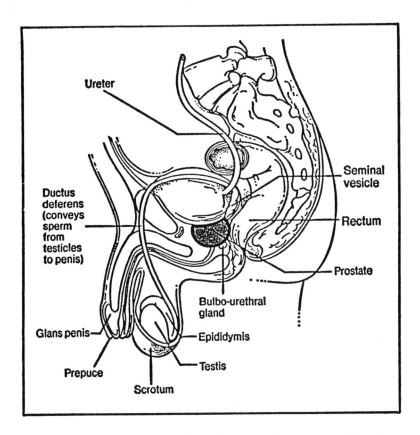

Ureter

Seminal vesicle

Ductus deferens (conveys sperm from testicles to penis)

Rectum

Prostate

Bulbo-urethral gland

Glans penis

Epididymis

Prepuce

Testis

Scrotum

Folk medicine has found several cures and pain-relievers for non-cancerous *orchitis*. The plant extract from *Echinacea* is especially effective against *testicular swelling*. Ten to 20 drops, taken hourly through the day, work well with nighttime mud packs to bring down swelling and take away pain. To keep the mud paste from drying out, add a tablespoon of *St. Johnswort oil* to the paste, or use a compress made from *squeezed cabbage leaves*. (If this causes a strong skin reaction, remove it immediately.)

Testicular Cancer isn't very common, but it is most likely to strike men between the ages of 18 and 32 and those over 60. Scientists have linked this to the thymus gland, which is very active in young men and suddenly becomes inactive at about age 60. Left untreated, *testicular cancer* can lead to death. But when it is detected early, it is 100 percent curable, doctors say.

The Spread of Testicular Cancer

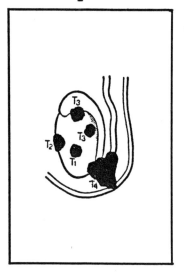 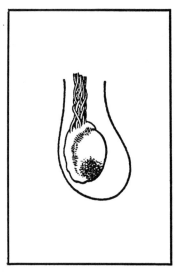

These two pictures show the eventual spread of testicular cancer if it is left unchecked. A quick, monthly self-examination can help a man to detect this cancer in its early stages when it can be successfully treated. The shaded areas show where the cancer most likely can manifest itself.

Every man needs to know how to perform a simple monthly self-examination for testicular cancer. The exam is easy, quick and very effective - and it could save your life.

INSTRUCTIONS
Self-exam for testicular cancer

Hold the testicles with both hands, being careful not to let them slip. Massage gently the entire surface of the testicles, checking for any hard lumps. Make sure you don't mistake the *epididymis* for a harmful growth - it is a soft, sausage-shaped "bump" that runs down the back of the testicles. The "wiry" texture within the *scrotum* is normal, too - it is the vas - the long tubes that carry the sperm away from the testes.

Should you feel any "knots," "pebbles," or "peas," or notice unusual puckers or "dents" in the skin, contact your doctor immediately.

Chapter 9

Natural Help For Prostate Cancer

Even with all the research and experiments going on, the average man with prostate cancer may want more options to choose from. There are unproven "cures" and plenty of "quacks" ready to prey on gullible or desperate cancer patients, but careful research will reveal that doctors and hospitals aren't the only places where relief can be found, if not a cure.

Even men who have no *prostate symptoms* - or a simple case of *prostatitis* - can benefit from many of the natural therapies outlined here. After all, today's healthy prostate may well fall prey to cancer as it ages. And as mothers say the world over: "An ounce of prevention is worth a pound of cure."

So even if it's too late for *prostate cancer* prevention, putting commonsense precautions into use could save you from developing cancer elsewhere in your body. Cut alcohol intake. Limit your exposure to the sun. Stop smoking, and avoid inhaling other smokers' fumes. Start an exercise program. Get regular checkups, and perform recommended self-examinations for mysterious lumps. Avoid environmental hazards like chemical fumes, dust or industrial pollutants.

It is also important to note that many "natural cures," thought in the past to be part of simple folklore, have been proven through laboratory tests to be directly beneficial to patients. Many medical doctors now prescribe treatments similar to those their grandparents used.

As I stated before, diet is the key to cancer treatment and prevention. Altering your intake of certain substances may work much like the immunotherapies prescribed by doctors - they build up the body's natural cancer defenses, or interfere with the chemical processes that cause cancer to spread.

Fiber and Prostate Cancer: The Seventh Day Adventist Study

Researchers at California's Loma Linda School of Medicine studied the diets and health of "normal" men against men who are observant Seventh-Day Adventists - a faith that prescribes a vegetarian diet. The researchers found the Adventists - who eat twice the amount of dietary fiber as the average men - had markedly lower incidence of *prostate cancers*. The researchers concluded that the vegetarians' low-fat and high-fiber diets help rid their bodies of excess hormone secretions, thus lowering their chances of developing prostate difficulties.

The study created a flurry of "high-fiber" diets and programs until another disproved some of its more extravagant claims. But a wise male will be sure to consume plenty of fresh vegetables and whole grains - thousands of healthy Adventist prostates can't be wrong!

Fruits, vegetables, berries, figs and dates are good sources of fiber, as well as brans and whole grains.

Fatty Acids: Omega-3 and Omega-6

A vegetarian diet is by definition a low-fat diet, another element that may contribute to freedom from cancer. Some researchers have linked human cancers to animal feed - almost all beef, pork and chicken raised for human consumption are fed artificial animal growth hormones to fatten them up and hasten their final trip to market.

Some researchers say these hormones remain in the meat - and act in odd ways on humans who consume them. No one has directly linked the animal hormones to human cancer, but it is a theory worth considering. Some prostate patients - some of them beef farmers - will eat only "free-range" or Kosher meat for this reason.

While a fat-laden diet may contribute to prostate cancer, it should not be confused with the body's need for essential fatty acids. Research discovered that *Omega-3*, a fatty acid abundant in fish oil, may be an effective cancer-fighter as well as a noted element in reduction of heart-attack risk.

Scientist studied the diets of Greenland, Iceland, Japan and Chinese populations whose diets revolve around their abundant fisheries. Almost none of the people suffered from *breast* or *prostate cancer*. When the study focused on people from the same ethnic groups who live and eat "Western-style," cancer incidence rose to average levels.

A study at Rutgers University and the Memorial Sloan-Kettering Cancer Center found that *fish oil* supplements reduced the size, weight and incidence of cancerous tumors in cancer-induced laboratory mice.

Humans are not mice. But ongoing studies support the *Omega-3* study, and show its beneficial effects at preventing cancer, if not helping alleviate its symptoms. The best available source of *Omega-3* is salmon. If availability or expense is an obstacle, *salmon oil* is also available in capsule form at health food stores.

Other essential fatty acids are associated with lessened prostate symptoms. *Linolenic acid* and *linoleic acid*, (*Omega-3* and *Omega-6*) found in *flaxseed* and *pumpkin seed oils*, are involved in production of prostaglandins - chemicals associated with sexual vitality.

Pumpkin seeds are used with success by many men who suffer BPH symptoms, according to *Nutritional Research News*. It is thought the seeds' concentrations of zinc, magnesium and phosphorus help decrease *prostate inflammation*.

Vitamin A: Hooray!

Researchers at the University of Arizona Cancer Center started another trend in 1982, when they announced they use Vitamin A as part of their anti-cancer arsenal.

Mark Bricklin describes their experiments in his *Encyclopedia of Natural Healing*: Mice injected with vitamin A responded remarkably better to radiation treatments than mice without the injections. Mice treated with only vitamin A or only radiation survived about two months after therapy ceased. Those treated with combination therapy survived 10 months, with less than 10 percent showing tumor regrowth.

Doctors have found positive links between intake of vitamin A and a lessened incidence of lung cancer in men. A comprehensive prostate cancer study undertaken in Japan revealed a substantially lower death rate from prostate cancer among men who ate green and yellow vegetables each day. Japanese scientists theorized that its the carotene — vitamin A — in these vegetables that my be responsible.

Food rich in carotene include carrots, sweet potatoes, squash, spinach, broccoli, pumpkins, kale and sweet red peppers. Studies in Wisconsin and Scotland found that even those cancer patients in relatively good health whose vitamin A levels were lower than average did not respond as well to chemotherapy as patients whose diets were rich in carotene.

The American Cancer Society estimates that dietary factors comprise 35 percent of Americans' cancer risks. Smoking contributes another 30 percent, and alcohol use another 3 percent. These elements are all under the control of individuals - and changing one's bad habits in regard to any of these elements can drastically cut cancer risks.

Foods Rich in Vitamin A

5 oz. sweet potato	15,000 IU
2 to 3 apricots	15,000 IU
1 cup peas and carrots	15,000 IU
1 cup baked butternut squash	13,000 IU
1 raw carrot	5,000 IU
1/2 mango	4,800 IU
1/4 cantaloupe	3,500 IU
1 stalk broccoli	3,500 IU
1 raw tomato	1,800 IU
1/3 papaya	1,750 IU
1 cup asparagus	51,500 IU

IU = International Unit

Carbohydrates and Fats

The National Cancer Institute advises Americans to keep their total fat intake to less than 30 percent of their diets, and to increase intake of complex carbohydrates.

So where to begin? Start with fruits and vegetables. They are an ideal source of complex carbohydrates as well as a great source of vitamins and minerals. Complex carbohydrates are a natural aid to dieters, as they produce a filled-up feeling without a huge calorie load. They are also a natural energy source.

Don't confuse complex carbohydrates with simple carbohydrates - a man-made byproduct of refining and processing natural foods. Commercial white sugar, white bread, potato chips and corn chips are good examples of how man takes an excellent product of nature and crushes, dyes or fries it into a nutritional nightmare.

If you are fond of potatoes, eat yours baked, topped with a little broccoli and melted mozzarella cheese. You'll be surprised at how filling it is, and for less than 225 calories. Complex carbohydrates and fibers should be balanced with dairy products and protein for a balanced nutritional intake. It's not difficult to choose low-fat dairy products instead of their high-calorie counterparts. When choosing a protein source, choose lean cuts of meat, or better yet, poultry, fish, beans, peas or tofu.

Simply concentrating on eating lots of complex carbohydrates, and fiber and fewer dairy products and proteins, you'll see the hidden payoff - a diet that is lower overall in fat. You'll feel satisfied with fewer calories.

Cornell University researchers tested the effects of such a diet against other eaters on high- and medium-fat diets.

Those on the lowfat diet ate as much food as they wanted, but consumed 627 fewer calories than their counterparts.

A Macrobiotics Diet for Prostate Cancer

Back in 1975, Mr. M. was diagnosed with prostate cancer. He was in his mid-50s.

Despite undergoing conventional treatments under his doctor's direction, the cancer spread into his spine, hip and shoulder.

Surgery was performed to remove a portion of one testicle, and radiation and chemotherapy were administered. Mr. M. also took hormone therapy pills, but his outlook continued to dim. Chemotherapy was particularly hard for him. His pain continued, and he vomited for up to 12 hours after each treatment.

By 1980, he'd had enough of chemotherapy. He agreed to continue the hormone treatments, though - and consulted with a doctor who recommended he try a macrobiotic diet.

Mr. M. noticed results almost immediately. His appetite and energy returned. In a month's time he was able to cut his hormone consumption in half, and after six months his doctor discontinued it altogether - the pain was gone.

M. knew intuitively, by the way his body felt, that he was well along the way of conquering his prostate cancer. He decided to confirm this feeling by having a bone scan done - an X-ray view of his skeleton. M. and his doctor both did a double take when the films came back. The malignancy had shrunk considerably. The shoulder, spine and hip were clear of the dark shadows of cancer that had previously appeared there.

As you may imagine, M. is now an enthusiastic

supporter of the macrobiotic way of life. "I am totally convinced that we are what we eat," he says, 13 years after that bone scan was completed. "We literally destroy our bodies with the poor-quality foods we consume."

M., now well into his sixties, still works full-time, frequently putting in more than eight hours each day. "I maintain a reasonable amount of exercise and look on cancer as something we can overcome with diet and determination," M. explained. "We have amazing bodies. They can heal themselves if we furnish them with the proper nourishment and eliminate the harmful."

M.'s healing discovery comes from the Orient, where human culture traditionally lives in harmony with nature. Macrobiotics is a method of extending life and conquering disease - including cancer - by consuming food derived from one's immediate environment.

Before the days of refrigerated shipping and worldwide food imports and exports, everybody ate macrobiotic diets. Those who lived on the plains of Africa and America ate plenty of grains, fruits and the occasional serving of wild meat. Eskimos consumed fish and high-fat preserved meats, which helped them conserve body heat. Each society ate a diet very different from the other, but each provided the nutrients their environments demanded for human survival.

Chinese, Korean and Japanese groups adopted and adapted the macrobiotic diets of their ancestors, and passed the dietary practices on to their children.

In more recent years, Micho Kushi, a Chinese nutrition consultant, refined the ancient macrobiotic concept to match the needs of modern Americans. His diet is designed to provide a perfect balance of nutrients required by healthy cells. These foods assist the body's natural elimination of built-up toxins, fats and mucus - all of which clog the tissues and cells and lead to disease.

The standard macrobiotic diet is heavy on whole grains, beans and cooked vegetables, along with certain supplementary foods, drinks and oriental condiments. Ideally, most of the vegetable and grain items should be grown within 50 miles of home - the very best are those grown in your back yard garden!

Fifty to 60 percent of each meal should be *whole* grains: *brown rice, oats, corn, barley, buckwheat* and *millet.* Another 25 to 30 percent should be *fresh* vegetables like *cabbage, carrots, turnips and their tops, onions, squash, cauliflower, Swiss chard, bok choy, watercress, burdock root* and other, locally-grown produce.

Eat up to a third of your vegetables raw, in salads. Kushi warns, however, that those suffering from cancer should be careful to limit their intake of raw foods, and should cook their vegetables before eating.

Vegetables high in acid or fat should be excluded from a macrobiotic diet. They include: *tomatoes, eggplant, potatoes, asparagus, spinach, yams, beets, zucchini, avocados and peppers.*

Beans and sea vegetables are an important element of macrobiotics, too. Recommended lowfat beans are: *lentils, chick peas and azuki beans.* Mineral-rich sea vegetables *like hiziki, kombu, wakame, nori, seaweed and Irish moss* are available at health food stores or Oriental markets. They can be eaten as a side dish or added to soup.

Soup consumption, however, should be limited to two small bowls per day. It should be prepared with recommended beans, vegetables or whole grains, and should always include some wakame seaweed, experts say.

The diet allows drinks like cereal-grain coffees, spring water drunk at room temperature, teas made from roasted barley, brown rice, or bancha twigs, and dandelion tea.

This is only a small taste of the macrobiotics diet. Some say its wondrous effects are due to the trained specialists who tailor each diet to the needs of the patient. These dietitians are available at local chapters of the East West Foundation, which supplies referrals, nutrition counseling, cooking classes and courses on macrobiotic philosophy.

For information write their national headquarters:

The East West Foundation
17 Station Street
Brookline, Massachusetts 02146
(413) 623-5741

An Austrian "Naturopathic" Treatment for Prostate Malignancy

The Austrians look to herbs to help them deal with prostate cancer. Several of the herb tea recipes provided in previous chapters will give prostate cancer patients needed relief of symptoms while medical treatments are tried.

Please note that these diets are not meant to treat or cure cancer or any other prostate complaint - they are supplements to a doctor's care, NOT substitutes.

The Austrian naturopath *Rudolph Breuss*, who created the treatment below, is credited with preventing and even curing a wide range of cancers, including *prostate cancer*.

He, too, testified to the effectiveness of the *small-flower willow herb*. Patients should sip two cups of cold tea each day, made by simmering a pinch of willow herb in a pint of hot water.

He also suggested a *3-week regimen* of "kidney tea," an herbal mixture that cleanses and soothes the urinary tract.

INSTRUCTIONS
Kidney Tea - 3 weeks' supply

Mix together:
   15 grams Horsetail
   10 grams nettle (best picked in Spring)
   8 grams bird knot grass (*polygonum aviculare*)
   6 grams St. Johnswort

Brew: Place of pinch of the mixture in a cup of almost-boiling water. Allow to steep for ten minutes, then strain. Add two cups of hot water and boil for 10 minutes, strain again.

To Use: Drink a half cup of this tea, cold, first thing in the morning; before lunch and again before bed. **Take for three weeks only.** Wait another two or three weeks, then resume. Do not eat meat broth, beef or pork while on this regimen.

Normal urination should resume after three days of starting the kidney tea.

Kidney tea is only part of this doctor's "total cure for cancer." This philosophy holds that a cancer tumor is an autonomous growth, and can only be eliminated by fasting combined with a juice and tea therapy. Although the regimen

* DO NOT use any form of sugar during this 42 day fast for cancer treatment in teas, or elsewhere. IMPORTANT

is rigorous, most patients don't lose much weight. Recipes for two other important herbal teas in this treatment are given below.

INSTRUCTIONS
Sage Tea
Place one or two teaspoons of sage in a pint of water and boil for three minutes. Add a pinch of St. Johnswort, lemon balm and peppermint. Steep for ten minutes, then strain.

Cranesbill Tea (*geranium robertianum*)
Cut very fine a large stem of geranium robertianum, enough to make one full tablespoon. Add to one cup of very hot water, steep for 10 minutes. **Drink cold. Do not add sugar to either tea.**

The 42-day cancer treatment limits patients to recommended teas and a special vegetable juice. The juice satisfies hunger pangs, but patients should be careful to drink no more than a pint per day of the vegetable mixture. **The juice must be taken by the spoonful, slowly, so it mixes with saliva before swallowing.**

INSTRUCTIONS
Vegetable Juice Mixture
Combine in a juicer or food processor:

    3 parts red beets
    1 part carrots
    1 part celery
    1 small radish
    1 egg-size potato   *continued...*

---

* DO NOT use any form of sugar during this 42 day fast for cancer treatment in teas, or elsewhere. IMPORTANT

INSTRUCTIONS
Vegetable Juice Mixture *continued*

Use a juicer to liquefy the vegetables.

NOTE: If the potato taste spoils the mixture for you, you can omit it here and instead drink a cup of potato peel tea each day. Put a handful of potato peelings in a pint of water and boil for 2 to 4 minutes.

SUGGESTED DIET ROUTINE

Upon waking: Half cup of cold kidney tea, sipped slowly.

An hour later: One or two cups sage tea.

An hour later: Small mouthful of vegetable juice.

Half hour later: Small mouthful of vegetable juice.

Lunchtime:
10-15 mouthfuls vegetable juice.
Sage tea, unsugared.
Half cup cold kidney tea.

Afternoon:
Mouthfuls of vegetable juice as needed.
Sage tea, unsugared.
One cup cranesbill tea.
Half cup cold kidney tea.

After the 42-day regimen ends, slowly begin to eat light solid food again - nothing heavily salted. Continue to drink about half a cup of vegetable juice each day before meals for two to four weeks. Augment the treatment with light exercise and plenty of fresh air.

* DO NOT use any form of sugar during this 42 day fast for cancer treatment in teas, or elsewhere. IMPORTANT

Naturopaths believe this cancer "cure" will not work on smokers who continue their habit.

Those coping with a *prostate cancer* problem will do well to review the herbal relievers listed in chapter 5. Whether the swelling and pain rises from *cancer* or *BPH* or *prostatitis symptoms*, herbs like the *small-flower willow* or *Damiana* are proven to provide welcome relief.

A Natural Alternative to Constipation

One simple reliever for prostate cancer pain - or simply the pain of a swollen gland - is keeping your bowels clear. Constipation can add to the abdominal congestion caused by bladder and prostate complaints, making a bad situation downright miserable.

Constipation is defined as "the abnormally delayed or infrequent passage of dry, hardened feces." It is important to understand that a bowel movement is not necessarily "abnormally delayed" if one doesn't occur naturally every day. Every body is different, some need to "go" once or twice daily, others only evacuate their bowels every other day or so. When the digestive tract is functioning properly, the body maintains its own rhythm and doesn't require a stimulant laxative.

Sadly, the discomfort, embarrassment and pain of constipation symptoms are a way of life for many. Long-term constipation has been linked to other maladies like *varicose veins* and *hemorrhoids* - even *high blood pressure*.

Aside from organic causes like *spastic bowel syndrome*, *tumors* or *diverticulitis*, much constipation occurs because of bad bowel habits. Normal intestinal function demands we allow the bowels to move when they will - a lower intestine can fill up in less than six hours. However, through habit, many have trained their bodies to retain waste for 24 hours or more. When nature calls, the urge should be answered quickly, to avoid developing bad bowel habits that may lead to constipation.

The German "Handbuch für Männer mit Prostataleiden" ("Handbook for Men with Prostate Problems") says constipation worsens cooperative functions of the bladder and its emptying muscle. When you are constipated, the increased volume of your bowels puts pressure on the pelvic organs. Common cholesterol buildup adds even more pressure to the stressed region. Symptoms like shivers and chills sometimes result - a condition the German text calls "cold constriction." The bladder muscle tightens up because of the body-wide chill, and thus constricts urine flow.

Bladder and bowel complaints also result from too much heat. Upholstered furniture, too many sweaters and over-heated rooms can raise the internal body temperature and over-relax internal muscles - including the bladder. Extended exposure to heat can make internal muscles slack and flabby. This German medical text simply states that the old rule of "moderation in all things" applies to temperatures, too, and warns men that *bare feet* and *cold drafts* can lead to *illness* later on.

I have already covered the importance of fiber in a healthy diet. High-fiber foods contain no calories and benefit the bowel by aiding digestion and keeping food by-products from collecting in the bumpy-textured surface of the lower intestine. Other substances are required to "keep the pipes clear," not the least of these being plenty of water throughout the day - up to eight 8-ounce glasses.

But what NOT to do for constipation is just as important as what you do to relieve it. The first impulse when this condition strikes is to reach for a laxative - more than $100 million is spent each year on laxatives and cathartics. There are about 5,000 types of bowel evacuents on the market - some of them are harsh or even poisonous substances that can cause as many problems as they cure.

Mineral Oil is the bugaboo of the laxative world - the American Medical Association has been preaching against its use for 30 years. Although it is an obvious lubricant, it decreases the body's ability to absorb calcium and phosphorus from food. The *mineral oil* itself absorbs vitamins A, D, E, K and carotene from the nutrients in the intestines, and takes fat-soluble vitamins and minerals from tissues throughout the body. All these valuable substances are then excreted and lost.

Stimulant laxatives like *castor oil* and the chemical *phenolphtalein* work directly on the small intestine to purge out any food matter. These are frequently prescribed by doctors for use prior to medical tests, and their occasional use is not harmful. But frequent purges can cause excess loss of water and body salts, resulting in body weakness. Many popular over-the-counter laxatives are of this type: too harsh for frequent use.

Saline laxatives like *Milk of Magnesia* and *epsom salts* produce rapid and complete results. The resulting bowel action is so complete, however, that the body may require several days to re-start its digestive processing, resulting in "rebound constipation."

Those who feel they must have at least one bowel movement each day may set themselves up for laxative abuse - creating an artificial dependence on laxatives to create a daily evacuation. Overuse of laxatives can lead to *dehydration, malnutrition symptoms, spastic colitis, stomach and bowel disorders and even chronic diarrhea.*

There are times when it is wise NOT to take a laxative. Avoid any use if *stomach cramps, nausea, vomiting or fever* are present. These could be symptoms of *appendicitis*. Stimulating your bowels with a laxative could result in rupture of the inflamed organ.

The best treatment for constipation is prevention. Some authorities believe that the most important health maintenance is done on the digestive tract - the body's supply line. Waste material not regularly evacuated from the body can accumulate, and the toxic by-products of putrefication can be carried by the blood and lymph to every part of the body. There is a strong link between cleanliness and health of the intestinal tract and the good health of the body as a whole.

Establishing normal intestinal "flora" (natural bacteria that aid in food breakdown) is of primary importance to establishing normal bowel movements. The following kitchen recipe for a *natural food-based laxative* provides a cleansing, revitalizing start to defeating constipation.

Natural Food Antidote for Constipation (enough for one person, 1-2 weeks)

1 cup whey powder
1 1/2 cups Brewer's Yeast
1 cup wheat germ
1/2 cup psyllium seeds
1/2 cup whole flaxseed
1/2 cup whole mustard seed (optional)

Mix all ingredients together in a large bowl till uniformly blended. Store in a plastic bag or Mason jar. *continued...*

Antidote for Constipation - *continued*

To use: Place 1 or 2 tablespoons of the mixture in a cup with the beverage of your choice - coffee, tea, milk, juice or water - and swallow slowly. Always rinse it down with a *second glass of your favorite drink.* Some users prefer to simply put a spoonful in their mouths and wash it down with *plenty of liquid.* Take before meals, one to three times daily. Allow a day or two for results - this is not a chemical blast, but a gentle food-based laxative.

My doctor father used this natural remedy in his practice to treat thousands of constipation cases. It is gentle and shows no negative side-effects, but is without fail a healthy way to evacuate the bowel and create a healthy "internal environment" for ongoing intestinal health.

All the ingredients for this constipation antidote are readily available at health food stores or co-ops.

New Finding for Prostate Cancer: The Essiac Story

Just before this volume went to press, a product known to help cure hundreds of cancer cases in Canada was made available to the general public through health food outlets.

Its modern use dates to the early decades of the 20th century, when a nurse named Rene Caisse drew thousands of hopeless cancer patients and plenty of medical controversy to her Ontario cancer clinic. Her claim to fame was a herbal therapy she called *"Essiac,"* a series of concoctions she made from a tonic recipe provided by an *Ojibwa Indian* medicine man.

Despite hundreds of documented cures, the Canadian medical establishment forbade Caisse to practice until she gave up her formula for intensive testing.

Caisse closed her clinic in 1942, but continued to quietly treat those who contacted her for help. A loophole in Canadian law allowed her to dispense the tonic when a patient's doctor gave consent. Rather than sell her healing knowledge to a medical establishment that might forbid its use, she chose to live a modest life, frequently providing her services free of charge to dying cancer patients. Many survived to sing her praises.

Before her death in 1978, Caisse passed on her secrets to a friend, Boston physician Charles Brusch. Before his retirement Brusch was a leading Boston clinician, medical researcher and personal doctor to President John F. Kennedy. Brusch himself had cancer of the lower bowel, which he said completely disappeared after he used Caisse's formula.

Caisse chose a powerful partner in Brusch. This distinguished doctor didn't hesitate to introduce unheard-of methods to his medical practice, setting trends in polio vaccination, free care for indigent patients and acupuncture, to name a few.

Brusch began administering *Essiac* to his patients in 1959. According to medical records, prostate cancer patient Wilbur Dymond took the formula for two months. During that time, all hardness in his prostate vanished. He no longer suffered excruciating pain during urination, Brusch reported.

Magazine and newspaper journalists investigated several false "essiac" formulas that came and went over the years. None were Caisse's own; all of them faded from the market. Finally, with Dr. Brusch's weighty influence, a series of clinical tests were performed using Caisse's recipes. Brusch and his associates learned to heighten and concentrate the medicine's effects, and collected hundreds of notarized testimonials to *Essiac's* curative powers.

Unfortunately, the American medical establishment refused to continue cooperating with Brusch's clinical trials unless Caisse gave other researchers her formula for further experiments. When she refused, they labeled *Essiac* "an unknown remedy" and consigned it to its former folk remedy status.

Dr. Brusch's updated formulations are now available in North American health products stores under the name of *Flor-Essence* and *Pro-Essence*. (Canadian Food & Drug Administration forbid use of the name *"Essiac"* because of copyright problems.) No prescription is needed to buy the formulas.

The *Pro-Essence* formula is made from Caisse and Brusch's specialized prescription for *prostate sufferers*. When the substance is absorbed into the system, the end result is a slow removal of systemic waste and toxins from the body through a gentle regulation of bowel and urinary tract functions. Prostate patients who experience painful urine retention frequently find their urine flow gradually increasing to normal. Those with abnormally frequent bathroom visits find themselves returning to a more normal schedule.

Pro-Essence doesn't just treat the *prostate*. Its makers say it helps almost any problem that involves *inflammation or enlargement of urinary organs* - in men and women. Its tonic effect boosts the immune system, a great help to those undergoing chemical and radiation therapies for cancer - as testified by Ed Florkoue of Calgary, Alberta. His notarized letter of testimony says the formula relieved his nocturia and dysuria during a long series of radiation treatments for his prostate cancer.

And for the elderly father of Cypriot-Canadian Elli Fletheriou, it proved a cancer cure. Mrs. Fletheriou wrote in a 1993 testimonial letter that her father was diagnosed in Oct. 1992 with a growing prostate cancer. He began taking *Pro-Essence* immediately, and took two bottles along when he went to Cyprus a month later to visit relatives. Three months later, he reported to a Cypriot oncologist for a "tumor checkup." But digital, PSA and needle biopsy tests both found no evidence of cancer.

"We were overwhelmed with surprise at the fast results," Fletheriou wrote. "I still can't believe *(Pro-Essence)* worked so fast on my father, who, by the way, is not a very good keeper of health or diet regimens."

Harold Good, a 75-year-old man from Vancouver, Canada, told an investigative reporter from *The Vancouver Sun* about the effectiveness of this cure on his prostate problems.

Harold had grown used to rising hourly throughout the night to urinate, "a painful and exhausting ritual," as he termed it. After his wife, Peggy, experienced a seeming miraculous cure from ovarian cancer using an *Essiac* formula, he decided to try it.

He went to bed early one evening, and rose a few hours later "in a sleep-walk" to relieve himself. Peggy visited the bathroom a few minutes later and was astonished at the gruesome discharge her husband had left behind in the toilet bowl.

"It was a bowl full of pus," she told the reporter. She went to wake Harold, to tell him something was wrong, but he was fast asleep. That was his last late-night bathroom excursion. His prostate hasn't troubled him since, he said.

Elaine Alexander, current holder of the secret formula, admits its primary ingredients are *slippery elm bark, burdock root, sheep sorrel and turkey rhubarb root.* Only Alexander and Brusch now know the correct harvesting, handling and decocting method.

Dr. Jim Chan, a Vancouver naturopath who teaches at a Seattle medical college, says burdock root contains *inulin,* a powerful immune-system modulator. He has used Alexander's tonics to treat cancer patients, but cautions against anyone believing they are the cure-all for cancer. He says they work best for patients who've had minimal radiation or chemotherapy treatments, and their effectiveness varies from patient to patient.

Caisse herself never claimed to have a sure cancer cure, but her legacy of living patients speaks for itself, Alexander says.

Like many other powerful medicines, *Pro-Essence* and *Flor-Essence* have a healing history traceable to indigenous people. Caisse said she obtained a crude recipe for *Essiac* from a patient who, in her youth, had treated cases of breast cancer with it. The patient got the remedy in the forest of northern Ontario, from an Ojibwa medicine man. All the herbs contained in the formula are native to Ontario.

There is hope for the hopeless, it would seem, if the testimony of Dr. Brusch is to be believed. As he wrote in his clinical findings: "The results we obtained with thousands of patients of various races, sexes and ages, with all types of cancer, definitely prove *Essiac* to be a cure for cancer. Studies done in the United States and Canada also fortify this claim."

Chapter 10

Impotence: A Man's Secret Nightmare

"About 1 out of every 10 men in the United States, from teens to senior citizens, suffers from chronic or continuous impotence." - Greater Pittsburgh Impotence Center

Impotency. The word conjures up nothing but negative associations - and fear that one's sex life is gone forever. Medical authorities define impotency as "the continued failure of a man to achieve and sustain an erection adequate for penetration of the female vagina."

Sex researchers Masters and Johnson describe a man as impotent when his "failure rate approaches 25 percent of his total sexual attempts."

Just look at the words used, all items that strike at the very base of the male ego: *"Failure* to *achieve* or *sustain."*

Inadequate. Unable to achieve. Continued failure. What man would admit to such a condition?

Unfortunately, the vast majority of those men whose prostates are surgically removed or irradiated by radiation are rendered impotent. "Nerve-sparing" prostatectomies preserve potency, and are becoming more widespread. But it seems anytime a man's reproductive organs are affected by illness, impotency can be at least a temporary problem.

Sometimes impotence happens when a man simply believes his treatment will make him impotent. In these cases, even when doctors find his "equipment" perfectly intact and functional, the man cannot get an erection.

Before a man concludes he is impotent, he should understand the many outside causes that can interfere with erections. Impotency can be traced back to use of certain medications and prescription drugs, high stress levels, alcohol, disease or family problems.

Another cause is some mens' unrealistic view of their sex drives. As a man ages, his body reacts differently to sexual stimulation. He may take longer to become aroused and achieve an erection. A 55-year-old whose standard of virility is the average teenage male is bound to be disappointed in his own performance. Many men don't realize their slowed reactions are natural body changes. They mistakenly believe they are growing impotent. But before I go into the changes you can expect, it's important you know just how an erection works.

More Anatomy

The penis is made of three parallel cylinders, enclosed in an outer sheath of stretchy, elastic skin.

The two major cylinders, called the *corpus cavernosum*, are responsible for the bulk of an erection, and provide the erection's familiar rigid, firm shape. These two cylinders of spongy tissue may be compared to long balloons. When pumped full of blood they are erect; when not, they are small and limp.

The Penis

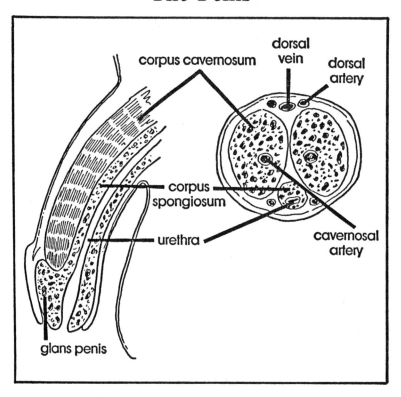

corpus cavernosum

dorsal vein

dorsal artery

corpus spongiosum

urethra

cavernosal artery

glans penis

From *"BioPotency: A Guide to Sexual Success,"* by Richard E. Berger, M.D., and Deborah Berger, M.S.W., Rodale Press.

The inside of these cylinders is lined with millions of tiny sponge-like caverns called "sinuses." They fill with blood during arousal, but when the penis is flaccid, only enough blood for cell maintenance is present. Millions of tiny sphincters close and open according to incoming stimuli - a complex, intricate system that functions entirely without conscious thought on the male's part. Erection is an involuntary response. Even though some women may not believe it, a man cannot "will an erection."

The third cylinder, called the *corpus spongiosum*, surrounds the urethra - the channel through which semen and urine travel to the outside world. This cylinder also fills with blood during an erection, but it doesn't take on the firmness of its two neighbors. It has another important function to perform.

The *corpus spongiosum* is connected to the *glans penis*, the tip or head of the penis - the organ's most sensitive spot. Those all-important nerves that provide sexual sensation are located here, and travel through the *corpus spongiosum* to the spinal cord, which gives erection its "reflexive" character. (So is proven the old adage: It doesn't take any brains to get an erection!)

Mental stimulation results as sensations travel to the brain. All these signals pass back and forth through the *pudendal nerve*, one of a bundle of nerve fibers that lies along the *corpus spongiosum*.

Two other sets of nerves: the *sympathetic and parasympathetic nerves*, control ejaculation and erection, respectively. When sexual arousal becomes intense enough that climax is inevitable, a message travels from the brain down the spinal cord to the sympathetic nerves. This message tells the muscles around the base of the penis to contract rhythmically and release the semen.

Male orgasm is composed of two phases: emission and ejaculation. During sexual arousal, sperm is pumped from the *scrotum* (which encases the testes), through the vas and into the region around the *ejaculatory ducts*. The longer the period of foreplay before climax, the more semen is pumped into the ducts. Emission is the moment called "ejaculatory inevitability." This is when the *seminal vesicles* behind the prostate gland contract and release the seminal fluid.

Ejaculation happens soon afterward, when the muscles surrounding the base of the penis contract powerfully at about one second intervals. The semen is pushed out of the penis with great force. Thus, emission is the collection of seminal fluid and sperm, while ejaculation is its elimination. Once emission occurs, it is impossible to voluntarily delay ejaculation.

What Can Go Wrong
Tiny Veins and Squeezing Sinuses

The rigidity, or stiffness, of an erection comes from an extra spurt of blood into the *corpus cavernosum*. Important arteries supply blood to the "sinuses," which expand and stiffen the organ.

The Penile Sinuses: Before Erection

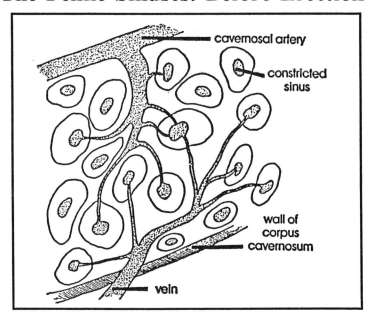

The sinuses are constricted and contain only a small
amount of blood when penis is flaccid.

The Penile Sinuses: During Erection

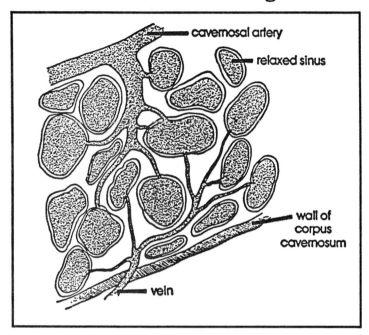

The blood flow increases and the sinuses expand, compressing the veins, when the penis is becoming erect.

From "BioPotency: A Guide to Sexual Success," by Richard E. Berger, M.D., and Deborah Berger, M.S.W., Rodale Press

Tiny thin-walled veins drain blood away from the *sinuses* after climax. These veins are more important than doctors once thought: Dr. Tom Lue, a University of California urologist, has demonstrated that the expanding *sinuses* compress these veins and slow the blood flow out of the penis. But if the veins aren't squeezed tightly enough during erection by the expanding *sinuses*, blood flowing to the penis will simply flow back out through these veins, resulting in either a poorly sustained erection or none at all - much like trying to fill a bathtub without first closing the drain.

There are reasons why these veins may not work properly:

1. Not enough blood is getting to the sinuses. They are not swelling enough to cut off the veins' draining effect.
2. The sinuses are too stiff to be expanded by the incoming blood.
3. The veins are abnormally formed at birth, so they cannot be squeezed shut.

None of these are reason enough to resign yourself to a life of celibacy. Any of them can be successfully treated by a specialist.

Fear

Because erection is such a complicated process, many factors can be involved in its failure. Probably the largest factor is fear. A man's "performance anxiety" can actually influence his sexual ability. John P., a man happily married for 12 years and father of three children, is a good example.

John's wife Ellen experienced a number of health problems that prompted her doctor to advise against any more pregnancies. He suggested Ellen undergo a *tubal ligation*, or John a *vasectomy*.

John, a generous man, felt his wife had undergone enough medical probing. he volunteered to undergo a *vasectomy* in order to "give Ellen a break from the hospital."

John knew vasectomies don't cause impotency - it simply sterilizes the man through removing the *vas deferens*, the path through which sperm travel from the *scrotum*.

But John's father, who had also undergone the surgery, warned his son he was "never the same after that operation."

He never fully explained what he meant. John, though, concluded he must have meant impotency.

John went through with the surgery, despite his misgivings. And after he recovered, he could not get an erection. He had convinced himself, with the help of his father, that he "would not be the same" after the operation.

After two months of therapy, John and Ellen resumed a normal sex life. But not without finding out what a powerful enemy fear can be to a healthy lifestyle.

Even after an erectile problem is "solved," fear of later failure may haunt a man, setting him up for further disappointments and creating a "self-fulfilling prophecy" of failure.

It's All In Your Head

The brain is man's most potent sex organ. Men can get easily aroused through visual stimulation, but his fear of not being able to perform can lead to erectile problems.

Researchers believe a chemical found in the brain is vital to a man's sex drive. It is called *acetylcholine*, and supposedly triggers the sex organs' initial reactions to stimuli. If there is a lack of this chemical in the brain, a man rarely thinks of sex and, in fact, will not be stimulated through visual means.

The body makes *acetylcholine* with certain dietary elements - primarily those found in seafood. Those who eat few fish and shellfish might consider a supplement like lecithin, which contains acetylcholine. *Lecithin* is available in several forms in health food stores. Authorities recommend about 7,200 milligrams a day for healthy males.

Lecithin is also good for the circulatory system. It breaks cholesterol down into particles small enough to leave the body. If cholesterol cannot escape, it remains in the blood and coats the insides of arteries, literally clogging the blood flow.

Because a man's erection depends on the free flow of blood to his penis, lecithin might be a suitable dietary supplement.

Age Changes Things

A man's response to sexual stimulation changes over the years. What some men consider a loss of potency is really only natural changes dictated by age. The changes in no way affect a man's ability to father children or the pleasure he derives from sex.

Sex researcher Kinsey reports a 2 percent impotency rate among 40-year-olds, 18 percent at age 60, and 25 percent at age 65. Another study reported a 31 percent impotency rate in the 55 to 59 age group.

The younger a man is, the easier and quicker he can achieve an erection. Some men in their late teens and early 20s report they have almost continuous erections, sometimes cause for embarrassment. Jim, for example, recalls his college years.

"I'd be sitting in class with an erection - I'd sometimes have an erection all day long. And it could be embarrassing! You'd have to lose it before you could stand up." A man at his sexual peak - late teens and early 20s - can have intercourse two or three times during a single encounter.

As he matures into his 30s, a man's erection will be a little slower. This change, in fact, may produce in him a greater interest in foreplay, which is usually a welcome change where his partner is concerned. This man will usually take a little longer to reach orgasm. He may find it easier to control his ejaculation and prolong the pleasure of intercourse for himself and his partner.

The climaxes may be slightly less intense, and the quantity of ejaculate may be less. But most men at this age report a deepening enjoyment of sex as a form of lovemaking and intimacy.

As a man reaches his 50s and 60s, even more time is needed to attain a firm erection. This doesn't mean the man is losing his ability to make love. No one should panic when these changes become apparent. Foreplay simply becomes more essential. Often the penis will need to be caressed to achieve a full erection.

Older men do not respond to visual stimulation the way they did at age 18. George was 65 when he took his potency concerns to his doctor.

"Nothing happens down there," he told the doctor. "I used to be able to get "hard" just by looking at a pretty girl. My wife is still quite pretty, and in the past I've always been able to just look at her and get an erection. I'm still really attracted to her, but I look at her and nothing happens.I can watch her getting undressed; I feel excited, but my penis just lies there."

George's problem was solved with a little help from his still pretty wife, who was glad to help him with a little direct stimulation and the addition of magnesium, zinc and B-vitamins in his diet. Their doctor helped George to "get real" with his expectations: Erections on men his age don't have the texture, urgency or forceful ejaculation of youngsters'. But what they lose in texture they gain in staying power.

Probably the most noticeable and disturbing feature of the aging process is the increase in "latency periods" - the time between successive ejaculations. For some men in their 60s, it may be hours before they can attain another erection. While this may prevent intercourse during the interval, it may provide more time for other forms of sexual activity.

None of these changes should be interpreted as a sign of impotency. They are simply changes in the ways the male body responds to sexual stimulation. Taken in stride, they offer opportunities to broaden the kinds of pleasure one can receive from sexual relations.

Other Causes for Impotency
Medication

It's hard to find a man over age 40 who isn't on some kind of regular prescription medication. Prescription drugs can be potency-killers - especially those used to control high blood pressure. Some mens' sexual performance declines dramatically after they begin blood pressure medication, but many simply attribute the loss to "old age," never considering the effect the medicine may have.

Other drugs that commonly affect potency include *barbiturates, tranquilizers, reserpine, narcotics, antihistamines, antidepressants and amphetamines* - alone or in combination with other chemicals. Controlled substances like marijuana and *cocaine* - including *"crack"* - may also steal away potency. The obvious solution is to consult with your doctor. If your health permits, suspect drugs should be temporarily stopped or alternatives found.

Drugs That May Affect Potency

GENERIC NAME	BRAND NAME	GENERIC NAME	BRAND NAME

Blood pressure medicines/diuretics

Thiazides	Diuril, Esidrix, Hygroton and others
Spironolactone	Aldactone
*Hydralazine	*Apresoline
*Minoxidil	*Loniten
Methyldopa	Aldomet
Clonidine	Catapres
Reserpine	Serpasil, Sandril
Guanethidine	Ismelin
Bethanidine	
Phenoxybenzamine	Dibenzaline

Antidepressants

Nortriptyline	Aventyl
Amitriptyline	Elavil
Desipramine	Norpramine
Doxepin	Sinequan
Imipramine	Tofranil
Isocarboxazide	Marplan
Phenelzine	Nardil
Tranylcypromine	Parnate
Pargylene	Eutonyl
Furazolidone	Furoxone
Procarbazine	Matulane
Lithium carbonate	

Anxiety medications

Chlordiazepoxide	Librium
Oxazepam	Serax
Diazepam	Valium
Chlorazepate	Tranxene
Meprobamate	Miltown, Equanil
Tybamate	Tybatran

Major tranquilizers

Fluphenazine	Prolixin
Trifluoperazine	Stelazine
Prochlorperazine	Compazine
Mesoridazine	Serentil
Promazine	Sparine
Chlorpromazine	Thorazine
Thioridazine	Mellaril
Haloperidol	Haldol
Droperidol	Innovar
Thiothixene	Navane
Chloprothixine	Taractan

Drugs for irregular heartbeats

Disopyramide	Norpace
Phentolamine	Regitine
*Prazosin	*Minipress
Propanolol	Inderal
Metaprolol	Lopressor

* Least likely to cause potency problems

Drugs for bladder or bowel spasms

Propantheline bromide	Pro-Banthine
Atropine (usually used in combination w/other drugs)	

Drugs for Parkinson's disease

Biperidin	Akineton
Cycrimine	Pagitane
Procyclidine	Kenadrin
Trihexyphenidyl	Artane
Benztropine	Cogentin
Levodopa	Larodopa, Sinemet

continued

Drugs That May Affect Potency
continued

GENERIC NAME	BRAND NAME
Drugs for allergies and motion sickness (antihistimines)	
Dimenhydrinate	Dramamine
Diphenhydramine	Benadryl
Hydroxyzine	Vistaril
Meclizine	Antivert, Bonine
Promethazine	Phenergan
Muscle relaxants	
Cyclobenzaprine	Flexeril
Orphenadrine	Norflex

COMMONLY ABUSED DRUGS

Alcohol
Amphetamines
Barbiturates
Cocaine
Marijuana
Narcotics (such as heroin and morphine)
Nicotine
Opiates

GENERIC NAME	BRAND NAME
Miscellaneous drugs	
Cimetidine	Tagamet (for ulcers)
Clofibtate	Altromid-S (for high cholesterol and high fat in the blood)
Cyproterone acetate	(a hormone used to treat certain types of cancer)
Digoxin	Lanoxin (for heart problems)
Epsilon aminocaproic acid	Amicar (for abnormal bleeding
Estrogens	(female hormones used to treat prostate cancer)
Glucocorticoids	(hormones used to treat severe allergies, asthma and other breathing problms, arthritis, lupus and other diseases
Immunosuppressive agents	(agents sometime used to treat arthritis and lupus; used by transplant patients to prevent tissue rejection)
Indomethacin	Indocin (mainly for arthritis)
Methysergide	Sansert (for headache relief)
Metoclopramide	Reglan (for heartburn)
Metronidazole	Flagyl (for infections)
Phenytoin	Dilantin (for seizures)
Progestins	(female hormones used to treat certain types of cancer)

Source: *Drugs and Male Sexual Dysfunction.* American Urological Association Update Series. (Houston: American Urological Association, 1984).

If you take medication and are experiencing erectile difficulty, keep these considerations in mind:

- A variety of drugs can cause erection problems. Some drugs, including the new wave of antidepression drugs *(Prozac, Zoloft)* are too new to have been identified as problematic.
- Different men have differing degrees of sensitivity to drugs. One man may lose his potency to a certain medication, while another man on an identical dosage will maintain full functioning.
- Drugs interact with each other. A man may take a single drug and experience no problems, but when he adds another medication he may develop erectile problems.
- The body's tolerance for medication may change with time. A medication taken for years without effect may suddenly steal away potency.

Alcohol

Overindulging in alcohol can cause erectile difficulty. If the drinking is only occasional, the difficulty usually passes away with the intoxication.

But those who indulge may frequently find their reflexes and sensory ability impaired long-term. Orgasms are less intense, and sex loses its savor.

Alcoholics may find they have erection problems even when they are "on the wagon." A heavy drinker may even permanently impair his ability to make love. Alcohol can damage the testicles' ability to produce testosterone. The liver damage that accompanies alcohol abuse changes the way the body uses testosterone. This adds up to a decreased sexual desire and inability to achieve or maintain erection.

Many alcoholics who seek treatment for impotence are given hormone shots to increase their testosterone levels, but this therapy isn't always successful. Those whose metabolism is permanently impaired sometimes report mild breast development and a softening of facial hair: their bodies convert the testosterone into female hormones!

One or two drinks may increase libido by loosening inhibitions and lessening stress. But anyone interested in a long, healthy sex life is well advised to imbibe in spirits only moderately.

Smoking and Environmental Factors

Research is beginning to point the finger at cigarettes and cigars as a cause for male impotency. Evidence links smoking to *hardening of the arteries*, including those vessels vital to erection. When penile and *pubic arteries* harden and narrow, they are unable to expand enough to allow sufficient blood into the *corpus cavernosum* to cause erection.

In most men, this condition develops over many years. Smoking cigarettes today may not effect your sex life. But research indicates this may be the case for a few highly-sensitive men. Among these, smoking may indeed cause erectile problems before the arteries are damaged.

Secondarily, smoking can contribute to *bladder cancer*, which frequently requires surgery. Many bladder surgeries leave the patient impotent.

Doctors find that other environmental pollutants found in the workplace may effect patients sexually. People who work with toxic chemicals, thinners, lead and other heavy metals frequently report erectile difficulty.

Diabetes and Chronic Diseases

Impotency is a classic first symptom of diabetes, a common metabolic disorder that can wait until later in life to strike. Loss of sexual function may be due to a combination of blood vessel changes and disorders of the nerves that connect the penis to the spinal cord.

Dr. Isadore Rossman details its symptoms in *"Looking Forward,"* a text on aging. He says that failure to have erections during the night, on awakening or during masturbation indicates an organic basis for the impotency - it's not just psychological.

Rossman estimates up to 50 percent of male diabetics develop impotency. Damaged nerves prevent sexual impulses from being transmitted to the valves of the penis. Even with abundant sexual stimulation, the message cannot get through, the valves remain closed, and blood is unable to enter the penis and produce an erection.

Similar problems may be experienced by men with vascular and neural impairments not related to diabetes. These problems are sometimes difficult for doctors to detect, but are more obvious in men whose nerve pathways were affected by previous surgeries, head or spinal injuries. Degenerative nerve disorders like multiple sclerosis and spina bifida may also effect potency.

Those with chronic *fatigue syndrome, mononucleosis, heart disease* and *stroke, genital or venereal disease, high blood pressure* and *emphysema,* as well as *severe low back pain,* may also suffer from impotency.

Those with *neural* and *vascular disorders* are ready patients for modern and old-fashioned impotency cures detailed later in this chapter. But prevention is the best cure:

those at risk for diabetes - black men and anyone with a family history of the disease - should carefully control their intake of sugary and high-fat foods.

Depression

Chronic depression is common among men of middle and elder years - the time when unmet youthful expectations haunt the less-than-successful, and personal fulfillment issues plague those who've made it to the top. *Depression* wears away at sexual desire - its effect on *serotonin*, a brain chemical that regulates coping skills - is well documented. Depression may also throw off secretions of *testosterone* and *thyroid secretions.*

Counseling and a round of antidepressant medication may be required for relief. *Testosterone* may act as a supplement and a powerful placebo for some men whose self-doubts are augmented by sexual problems.

Endocrine Disorders

Your glands can take away your potency. The *thyroid, pituitary and adrenal glands* can all play roles in impotency. Talk about these with your doctor, and check your family's health history for relatives who may have suffered from too much or not enough of any of these secretions. Simple hormone imbalances may also effect potency.

Stress

Loss of a loved one or a job, finding a parking spot or getting a big promotion - all create their own forms of anxiety that can put the kibosh on sexual functions. Whether negative or positive, your body responds to these losses, responsibilities or almost any change with a rush of blood to the limbs - a good way to escape. The cumulative effect of these daily stresses can be impotence. Your blood is in your arms and legs, set to help you fight an enemy or run away. It's not in your central body, where it can easily flow "southward."

It may be impossible to eliminate some stresses, but if you learn to relax, slow down, say "no" to extra projects, you may find your sex life improving.

Determining the Cause

In recent years great strides have been made in diagnosis of impotency. Sometimes the cause is obvious - *prostatectomy, injury, birth defects or drug reactions* are easily detected.

Those with more "mysterious" ailments may undergo some of these diagnostic tests commonly used by doctors. This is only a brief outline, however; your doctor will have more detailed descriptions of his diagnostic tools.

Blood and Urine tests detect abnormal hormone, protein or body chemical levels that can indicate specific problems.

Cystoscopy is use of a special viewing scope to assess the bladder and prostate.

Corporacavernosogram is an X-ray method that frequently reveals conditions of restricted blood flow to the *corporum cavernosum* - the balloon-like erectile tissues.

Penile Arteriograms create a "map" of the blood vessels in and around the penis. Doctors can sometimes see blockages or damaged tissues and pinpoint where the problem lies.

Cystometrogram (CMG) or *Electromyogram* (EMG) are tests usually performed on the bladder. They test nerve and muscle functions that may influence the penis.

Bulbocavernosus Reflex Latency Time (BC Reflex) test and *Biothesiometry* indicate whether the penile nerve supply is normal for erection.

Nocturnal Penile Tumescence test (NPT) determines whether the cause of impotency is physical or psychological. The doctor uses a gauge or monitor to check the automatic erections every man has periodically as he sleeps. If these do not occur, the impotency probably has a physical cause.

What Can Be Done
Sex Therapy

Many impotency patients whose conditions were termed physical regained their sexual vigor through a standard course of sex therapy - sitting down and talking with a trained counselor, using visualization and relaxation exercises, and enlisting the help of a supportive partner. In a study cited by Dr. Anne Simons in her book "Before You Call the Doctor," a large group of men with "diabetic erection loss" were treated with a standard sex therapy course. Almost all regained their erections. Recent statistics give sex therapists an 80 percent success rating in treating erection problems.

Seeing a therapist doesn't mean you are mentally ill or somehow inferior. If you are ill, you go to a doctor to get better, don't you? Many of the therapy "exercises" are truly fun - one learns how to concentrate less on the penile sensations and generalize pleasure throughout the body through touching and sensual massage, just to name one option.

Yohimbine Therapy

If standard sex therapy doesn't work, the doctor may prescribe yohimbine, a drug derived from the bark of an

African tree with legendary aphrodisiac properties. About one third of the men who try this drug report increased erections, but its effectiveness seems to fade after a year or more of use. It works by stimulating blood flow to the penis.

Papaverine and Prostaglandin Injections

Many diabetics who are accustomed to injecting themselves with insulin make good use of *papaverine* - a "high octane" drug that is injected into the penis before sex. The drug relaxes penile blood vessels so more blood can get into the *corpus cavernosum*. *Papaverine* works within 10 minutes, and the resulting erection can last an hour or more. *Prostaglandin* is another vein-dilator in common use. Some men use these medications for years, but others shy away from their use, frightened at the prospect of wielding a needle in such a delicate area.

Vacuum Constriction Devices

One popular option is the vacuum constriction device, a plastic cylinder attached to a pump. The cylinder is placed over the flaccid penis before lovemaking, and the vacuum draws blood into the penis. A band is then put at the base of the erection, trapping the blood inside.

Almost 90 percent of the men who use these devices are satisfied with them. Manufacturers usually supply instructional videotapes and toll-free numbers to guide beginners.

But vacuum devices don't suit some others. Spontaneous sex is impossible, and the device is somewhat cumbersome to use, one therapist said.

Penile Implants

A surgical option chosen each year by about 25,000 men - a small minority is the penile implant, a surgically-installed prosthesis that makes the penis rigid enough for intercourse.

Some simpler implants are made of flexible, semi-rigid material - a permanent erection. Others are inflatable implants that are flaccid when not in use, but can be "stimulated" into erection through a squeeze bulb hidden in the scrotum.

The Inflatable Penile Prosthesis

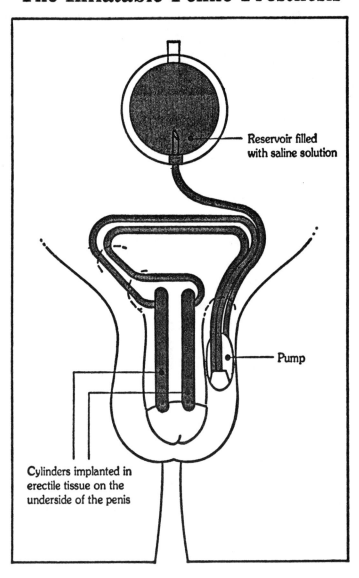

Reservoir filled with saline solution

Pump

Cylinders implanted in erectile tissue on the underside of the penis

Another "inflatable" uses hydraulic cylinders implanted in the penis. A fluid reservoir is placed in the abdomen, which provides a saline "filling" for the erection when the man pumps a squeeze bulb.

Hinged and "malleable" prostheses are also used by some doctors, but are waning in popularity.

Prosthetic implantation is a relatively simple surgery, requiring an hour or less under general anesthesia. Recovery takes two weeks or so, and sex can resume in four to eight weeks after surgery.

A Simpler Life

Some men opt to forego all the hardware and pharmaceuticals and simply learn to live with their impotence. They say they are just happy to be alive and cancer or pain-free, with or without sex. They find a fulfilling life through work, recreation and relationships that are free of sexual complications.

Chapter 11

Food and Supplements For a Richer Sex Life

Before you read or believe anything in this chapter, be aware that the federal Food and Drug Administration says there is no such thing as an aphrodisiac.

An aphrodisiac is a substance supposed to improve sexual vitality and performance. Laws expressly forbid manufacturers to make claims of sexual potency for their products, because their claims usually don't live up to the stringent pharmaceutical tests required by the FDA.

But man's centuries-old pursuit of bigger and better erections continues. The legendary attributes of some substances have produced some off-the-wall results: Poachers continue to deplete Africa's herds of white rhinoceros - in the Orient, the creatures' ground-up horns are believed to improve sexual performance. Other legendary "aphrodisiacs" include ground pearls, mandrake roots worn around the neck, ginger root tea, baths in special hot springs, and quarts of oysters, downed raw and chased with beer.

Let us take a moment to explore some of the world's more enduring stories of potent flora and fauna, in hope that some of the less exotic "aphrodisiacs" may have a grain of reality among the clouds of legend.

The Anango-Ranga, an Indian holy book, contains several recipes specially designed to increase male sexual vigor.

Some foods that appear repeatedly are *cucumbers, beans, sugar, asparagus, eggs, onions, garlic and honey.*

One recipe claims "the patient, no matter what his age, will retain vigor and be able to enjoy 100 women." The ambitious man should combine 150 grains of fiber from the *Moh tree (bassia latefolia)* with cow's milk, the Anango-Ranga says.

Scientists say the pith of the Moh tree contains up to 58 percent fermentable sugar - a ready source of energy. Honey would provide a good substitute effect.

Ginseng is another substance long touted for its sexual powers. Its scientific name *Panax Notoginseng* is derived from the Greek *Panax*, meaning "all-healing," and the Chinese *Schinseng*, meaning "man-root." The root of the *ginseng* plant sometimes resembles the human body. It is native to China, Korea and Siberia, but its most potent varieties grow wild in the United States.

Along with its aphrodisiac qualities the *ginseng root* is also credited with rebuilding tissues, stimulating energy and strengthening the body against mental and physical stress.

Ginseng isn't cheap, and it can be difficult to store while retaining its effectiveness. *Ginseng tea* is available in loose or bag forms at supermarkets, however, and stronger *ginseng drinks* can be found in most health markets and catalogs.

The Chinese have long believed that *Bird's Nest Soup* is a powerful aphrodisiac. The soup is traditionally made from the nests of sea swallows. They contain large amounts of mineral-laden edible *seaweed* and phosphorus-rich *fish spawn*.

Caviar, too, has been noted through history as a sexual stimulant. Legend holds that Empress Catherine the Great of Russia could not produce an heir with her husband, despite many attempts. She therefore ate several pounds of *caviar* and soon conceived. (She also employed the services of a captain of the Royal Guard, whose *caviar* consumption went unrecorded.)

But *caviar* is expensive, a luxury by anyone's standards. Few can afford to eat it by the pound. The following recipe makes a tasty spread for morning toast or an evening snack eaten on crackers. It contains only tablespoons of the "black gold," but some say that's plenty enough to stimulate the desired effect.

Potent Caviar Spread

2 tablespoons minced pimento
2 tablespoons anchovy paste
2 tablespoons minced chives or green onion
1 teaspoon lemon juice
3 tablespoons caviar

Mix thoroughly, refrigerate covered for at least 30 minutes before serving.

Those who still cannot stomach *caviar's* price tag may want to try *Herring Roe*, a less-expensive substitute, credited with creation of thousands of Russian and Ukrainian peasant children.

Herring Roe Spread

2 cans soft herring roe
1 ounce butter
2 sliced tomatoes
3 small fried potatoes
1/4 cup flour
4 slices cucumber
dash salt
2 slices toast

Roll the herring roe in the flour and fry lightly in butter. Sprinkle with salt. Serve on toast and top with cucumber and tomato slices; with the potatoes as a side dish.

Oysters are also legendary restorers of male potency. American railroad magnate and gourmand "Diamond Jim" Brady was said to have an enormous appetite for *oysters* on the half-shell - and for pretty actresses, too. This is a try-at-home recipe for those interested in exploring this option:

Oyster Bed Salad

2 dozen oysters, half-shelled or shucked
1 beet root, cooked and sliced
2 tomatoes, cut into chunks
1 cup raw carrot, grated
1/2 cup onion, sliced thin   *continued...*

Oyster Bed Salad - *continued*

1/2 teaspoon lemon juice (optional)
olives
salt and pepper to taste
4 large lettuce leaves

Arrange ingredients attractively on the lettuce leaves and sprinkle with lemon juice. If you prefer, cut up the lettuce and toss it in a bowl with other ingredients, using the lemon as a dressing.

Naturopathic doctors have discovered a few substances they say have direct and positive effects on sexual functions. A few are listed here:

Gotu-Kola -   A Chinese herb reported to be able to keep old age at   bay. Those who drink *gotu-kola* tea supposedly stay vital well into their 80s and 90s. The herb is a hormonal tonic. It has a soothing effect on the nervous system, and also aids in digestion, experts say.

Licorice -   This is not the black jujubes or whips sold at old-time movie houses, but a Chinese variation on the strong-flavored herb. Herbalists say the *licorice* plant contains more than 100 medicinal compounds. A legendary sexual stimulant, it is combined with milk and honey to boost male sexual desires. *Licorice* is also thought to be helpful in treating *high cholesterol, inflammations, wounds, fevers and allergies.*

Kava-kava - This is made from the root of *Piper Methsyticum,* a shrub native to the South Pacific islands. Natives scrape the roots and cut them into pieces, which are either chewed like gum or added to food. Consumed internally, *kava-kava* steps up the sex drive of men or women, the natives believe. Moreover, when *kava-kava* oil is spread on the tip of the penis, it controls premature ejaculation, natives say.

Sarsaparilla - The root of this plant, native to tropical America, has been said to contain *testosterone*, the hormone responsible for the human sex drive. Perhaps the movie cowboy who ordered a *sarsaparilla* soda in the Old West saloon wasn't such a sissy, after all.

A European Cure for the Impotent

Ongoing research in Europe has found that *O.K.A.S. Peptide*, a formulation of enzymes that encourage hormone production, is a useful tool in re-starting the sexual fire.

Elena Groth, a European naturopath who specializes in difficult cases of impotency, found a direct correlation between impotency and a man's unconscious sleep erections. Specialists have long suspected that hormonal imbalances play a vital role in impotency.

But Groth found that users of the *O.K.A.S. Peptide* formulation had nocturnal erections that lasted up to 50 percent longer than normal. She surmised that prolonged use of the formula slowly corrects hormone imbalances, which in turn normalizes erections. The effect works itself into the waking world, where a formerly impotent man can put the healing to use during sexual intercourse. Best results are obtained on men over age 50 who have suffered extended bouts of impotency.

Test results show this natural supplement has no noticeable side effects. It works well for men whose doctors can find no physical reason for their impotency. Light exercise seems to heighten the effects.

Joe H. was 49 when he decided to give up on sex - it wasn't worth the frustration and humiliation any more. For reasons no doctor could detect, he could not achieve an erection.

Joe's wife told him she would love him no matter what, but Joe felt robbed of a vital part of his manhood.

During a visit to his natural foods store for multivitamins, Joe picked up a trial bottle of *O.K.A.S. Peptide*, figuring he had nothing to lose in trying.

Within a month, Joe and his wife were able to make love again. His ego and feelings of self-esteem were restored as well, he said.

Hospital tests have shown *O.K.A.S. Peptide* is also effective in treating hormone variations in women, especially those experiencing troublesome menopause.

The formulation has the curious effect of stimulating the ovaries as well. Groth has had a measure of success treating cases of female infertility using *O.K.A.S. Peptide* in combination with other "female" herbs.

Because *Peptide formulations* are a bit expensive, many Europeans like to supplement them with *muira-puama*, an herb that seems to work in synergy with peptides, boosting their effectiveness.

Another unique healing combination from overseas is especially effective in cases where impotence is linked with prostate problems. It is a combination of *Beta Sitosterol, Campesterol* and *Stigmasterol,* all of which normalize prostate functions.

Sometimes called *"BCS,"* these natural ingredients can aid in prostate and impotency problems using an all-vegetable formula that is approved even for strict vegetarians. It is a proven cholesterol control, and works by suspending bile in the bloodstream and opening the bile duct and other glandular sphincters. It is now widely available on the United States health food market.

The Danes also contribute their bit toward the war on impotency with a herb and vitamin program called *"LV Therapy."*

This combination was developed by Flemming Norgaard, a Danish M.D. Patients who took his formula said *rheumatic pains, herpes viruses, angina pain* and "the tiring effect of old age" were relieved after a month or two of the supplement.

Norgaard said this isn't medicine: it's a food supplement that aids in cell growth and function. It contains several compounds I've already discussed, including *anti-oxidants, pumpkinseed, minerals, vitamin A* and several healing herbs. With its health-giving effects patients say their immune systems are strengthened. They get fewer colds, have more energy and better dispositions!

LV's happy effect on the urinary tract isn't the least of its powers. Taken regularly, it helps bladder and urethra disorders and keeps them from returning. It aids in curing even stubborn cases or incontinence.

Prostate sufferers also swear by *LV's* effectiveness, especially when used along with other cures. It normalizes prostate functions, and can help relieve stress and depression associated with disease or illness. The sense of well-being some men experience with its use can act as a natural aphrodisiac.

Damiana, a herb recommended for prostate relief, is truly a powerful aphrodisiac, according to Dr. Zofchak of Pennsylvania. He recommends taking the herb with *saw palmetto*, another natural substance that forestalls any irritation to the urinary tract and sexual organs.

Saffron, a bright-yellow, expensive herb from India, also is legendary as an aphrodisiac. Because it can be very dangerous in large doses, the editors of *Prevention Magazine* recommend taking *Riboflavin* supplements instead. Analysis of the *saffron flower* reveals high levels of this important vitamin, which aids in hydrogen transport among cells. It helps to break down fatty acids, and aids in removing toxins from nerve cells.

Many scientists believe that time-honored aphrodisiacs work on the simple *placebo* principal - if you believe it will work, it will. But most agree that the best sexual tonic is good health. Try a good, low-fat diet, plenty of sleep and light exercise, and see if that won't boost your libido!

Glossary

Acute   a condition with sudden onset of symptoms and a sharp rise in symptoms. Duration is usually short.

Androgens   hormones responsible for development and maintenance of male sex characteristics. Testosterone is an androgen. An absence of androgens will usually cause the prostate gland to shrink.

Atrophy   the wasting or shrinking in size of tissues or organs.

Balloon Dilation   a benign prostatic hypertrophy treatment also called transurethral dilation, it uses a catheter with a special balloon tip. While within the prostate, the balloon is inflated to enlarge the passage for urine flow.

Benign   a non-malignant growth that does not invade or destroy neighboring tissue.

Benign Prostatic Hypertrophy (BPH)   enlargement or growth of the glandular tissue of the prostate; typically begins around age 40. This is NOT cancer; it does not invade or attack neighboring cells. The condition may cause the prostate to grow against the urethra and compress the bladder outlet, causing voiding difficulty.

Biological Therapy   experimental medical cancer therapy based on boosting the body's own resistance to cancer. Substances under study include colony-stimulating factor (stimulates white blood cell production), and interferons and interleukins (body proteins that fight infection.)

Bladder   an elastic sac that stores the urine before it is removed from the body through the urethra.

Biopsy   removal of a small amount of tissue from an organ or gland for study and diagnosis. Most commonly used to determine if cancer is present.

Brachytherapy   a radiation therapy that uses implanted radioactive pellets or "seeds." Also called interstitial radiation.

Carcinogens   cancer-causing agents.

Catheter a hollow, flexible tube that is passed through the urethra into the bladder to drain off urine. Used during and after surgery, or whenever patient cannot urinate normally.

Chronic a condition that lasts or recurs over a long time. Some diseases are chronic because they progress slowly or symptoms persist for a long time.

Corpus Cavernosum two long cylinders located in the penis, which fill with blood and provide rigidity during erection.

Corpus Spongiosum a cylindrical channel that passes between the corpus cavernosum. It provides a channel for the nerve bundle that gives the penis tip its sensitivity.

Cystoscopy examination of the urinary tract through a special viewing tube; used to help find urinary obstructions.

Dysuria difficult or painful urination. Dysuria can be a symptom of prostate disorders.

Ejaculatory Ducts tubes that connect the seminal vesicles to the prostate and the urethra.

Ejaculation discharge or expulsion of semen from the penis, usually accompanied by an orgasm. The ejaculate fluid, or semen, consists of sperm and other secretions.

Epididymis   a long, convoluted tube that winds along the back edge of each testicle. Sperm are stored in the epididymis until they reach maturity.

Erection   enlargement and stiffening of the penis as a result of sexual stimulation.

Essential Fatty Acids   Nutritional acids that help maintain the elasticity of cell tissues.

Estrogen   a general name for female hormones, which are responsible for development of reproductive organs and secondary sex characteristics in females. Once used for prostate cancer treatment.

Fertile   capable of conceiving children.

Flow cytometry   a procedure used to measure the amount of genetic material within a biopsied cell sample. These samples help doctors plan cancer treatments.

High-energy radiation   a therapy that uses radiation accelerators like neutrons, protons and helium ions to irradiate cancer growths.

Hormone Therapy   a prostate cancer treatment that uses female hormones to reduce production of testosterone, which is needed for prostate cancer reproduction.

Hyperthermia   another word for "heat." Hyperthermia therapy uses microwave heat, applied to the entire body or to a specific area, to shrink cancer cells.

Hypertrophy   excessive development or growth of an organ or gland.

Incontinence   inability to control bladder or bowel functions.

Impotence   inability in the male to achieve and maintain an erection sufficient for penetration of a female vagina.

Macrobiotics   a method of extending lifespan and avoiding disease through diet and lifestyle in harmony with the environment.

Masturbation   stimulation or manipulation of one's own genitals for sexual gratification.

Metastasis   spread of cancer cells to other, unaffected parts of the body.

Nephritis   acute or chronic kidney inflammation. Sometimes a result of stagnation of urine due to untreated prostate problems.

Nocturia   urge or need to urinate at night.

Nodule   a small mass of tissue or a tumor, generally malignant.

Oncogene therapy potential cancer therapy that replaces defective genes with healthy ones.

Orgasm the climax of the sexual act. It is accompanied by muscular contractions, release of tension and pleasurable sensations. In men, orgasm is usually accompanied by ejaculation. Orgasm may occur without erection.

Parasympathetic Nerves the system of nerves responsible for male erections.

Potency-sparing technique a variation on the radical open prostatectomy, in which the nerves and blood vessels responsible for erection are left in place. Doctors find this unfeasible when the tumor is large or has spread throughout the prostate.

Penile Prostheses implants placed in the penis which allow simulation of a natural erection. Usually used by men rendered impotent through illness, surgery, hormone or radiation treatments.

Penis the male sexual and urinary excretory organ.

Potency ability to achieve and maintain an erection sufficient for vaginal penetration.

Prostate Gland   a chestnut-sized gland located directly below the male bladder and surrounding a portion of the urethra. It secretes a fluid component of semen, which is expelled during ejaculation.

Prostate Specific Antigen   a blood protein produced by the growth of prostate cells. A PSA blood test can usually detect prostate cancer through measurements of this protein in the blood.

Prostatitis   acute or chronic inflammation of the prostate, usually caused by an infection, congestion or irritation.

Pudendal Nerve   nerves responsible for carrying sexual sensations from the penis to the spinal cord and then to the brain. These nerves are frequently cut during abdominal prostate surgeries.

Resectoscope   a surgical instrument inserted into the penis during transurethral prostatectomy. It "resections," or cuts away, the prostate tissue interfering with urinary function.

Retrograde   condition in which sperm goes backward into the bladder instead of being propelled forward and out of the end of the penis. This is frequently a harmless result of some prostate operations.

Selenium   a trace element needed to preserve cell elasticity and improve oxygen supply to the heart.

Scrotum   the external skin sac that contains the testicles.

Seminal Fluid (semen)   a thick yellowish-white fluid that contains spermatozoa. It is a mixture of secretions from the testicles, seminal vesicles, prostate and Cowper's Glands, designed to deliver healthy sperm cells to the female reproductive system.

Seminal Vesicles two folded glandular structures that lie against the lower rear of the bladder. They provide sperm with a high-energy milk sugar, a component of the semen.

Sigmoidoscope   a viewing instrument about 10-inches long. It is sometimes introduced into the anus as part of a rectal examination.

Sperm, or Spermatozoa   the male sex cell or gamete that carries the male genetic information and strives to fertilize the female ovum and create new life. It is a component of semen ejaculated from the penis.

Stent   a tiny tubular device made of surgical metal or plastic. Surgeons use this experimental implant to relieve prostate gland obstruction and shore up the neck of the bladder.

Sterile	unable to produce offspring.
Suprapubic/ Retropubic Prostatectomy	surgical procedures by which all or part of the prostate is removed through an abdominal incision.
Sympathetic Nerves	set of nerves in a male responsible for control of ejaculation.
Testicles	two male reproductive glands that are enclosed in the scrotum. The testicles, or testes, produce sperm and androgens.
Testosterone	a male hormone which triggers prostate growth and other sexual maturation at puberty. It also triggers the male and female sex drive. Doctors have found its presence promotes growth and spread of prostate cancer cells.
Transrectal Ultrasound	a diagnostic tool that uses sound waves to create a computer image of the prostate. A doctor inserts an instrument into the rectum that bounces sound waves off the prostate, revealing areas of abnormal growth.
Transurethral Prostatectomy	Surgical removal of prostate tissue using a resectoscope through the penis rather than an abdominal incision. Transurethral incision of the prostate (TUIP) uses a similar system to remove the core of the

prostate. Transurethral ultrasound-guided laster-induced prostatectomy (TULIP) uses ultrasound to guide the resectoscope and a high-energy laser beam to remove interfering tissue.

Tumor
a swelling or enlargement due to abnormal tissue growth. Tumors grow faster than neighboring tissues and serve no useful purpose. They can be benign (harmless) or malignant (cancerous.)

Uremia
a toxic excess of urine and other wastes in the blood. These wastes are usually processed through the kidneys. Uremia may be a symptom of prostate trouble.

Urethra
the muscular tube through which urine passes from the bladder and out of the body. In men, both urine and seminal fluid pass through the urethra.

Urine
waste fluid excreted by the kidneys, stored in the bladder and expelled through the urethra. Urine is 96 percent water and four percent dissolved waste substances.

Urology
the study, diagnosis and treatment of diseases of the genitourinary tract.

Vas Deferens
one of two tubes attached to the epididymis, extending to the prostate and loop-

ing upward behind the bladder. It carries mature sperm through several developmental steps and glands before delivering it to the urethra for ejaculation to the outside.

Zinc   a trace mineral essential for reproductive health. Zinc deficiency has been linked to prostatitis and impotency in men.

Appendix I:

Groups and Organizations That Can Help

No man need suffer alone when dealing with prostate problems, cancer or impotence. Many medical organizations, self-help groups and support services exist for the man or wife willing to take the first step.

Several studies show that men who seek support recover more quickly from surgery. Of those with cancer, a Stanford University study found that support group members lived an average of 36 months after joining the group. Men who didn't join usually lived about 18 months. Group members had a better outlook on life, doctors said, and were less moody, fatigued and depressed.

For up-to-date information on cancer, BPH, support groups and other information sources, start with your doctor; or one of the organizations listed below:

American Cancer Society
National Headquarters
1599 Clifton Road Northeast
Atlanta, GA 30329
(800) ACS-2345

American Foundation for Urologic Disease
1120 N. Charles St. #401
Baltimore, MD 21201
(800)242-AFUD

Provides referrals to local urologists; general information on urinary tract problems.

Cancer Information Service
(800)4-CANCER

These are cancer information specialists. They can provide free brochures on nutrition, metastasis, regional support organizations, prostate cancer research and radiation therapies - among dozens of others. Trained counselors can also tell you about clinical trials for prostate cancer, performed through the National Cancer Institute.

Impotents Anonymous
PO Box 5299
Marysville, TN 37802

Founded by diabetic impotence patient Bruce MacKenzie, this group helps the chronically impotent man regain his self-confidence and explore his options.

Local Hospital Support Programs

Most hospitals with cancer treatment units also provide patient support groups, educational seminars and informational meetings. Contact the social services department of your hospital, or ask your doctor for a referral.

National Cancer Institute
Office of Communications
Bethesda MD 20892

This federal institute offers a periodical prostate cancer research update. It can usually inform you on clinical trials that are taking place in your area.

National Council Against Health Fraud
PO Box 1276
Loma Linda, CA 92354

This non-profit group provides information on health frauds, quack cures and misinformation in public health systems. It produces a brochure on a lineup of "questionable" cancer cures. Some users, however, feel the group is unfairly biased toward medical and surgical treatments.

National Institute of Diabetes, Digestive and Kidney Diseases
part of the National Institutes of Health
Atlanta, GA.
(301)496-3583

Referrals usually available to local clinical trials in experimental treatments for BPH and prostatitis.

National Second Surgical Opinion Program Hotline
(800)23-SIMON

Call this toll-free number for free information on urinary incontinence.

Physicians Data Query (PDQ) at the National Cancer Institute

This is a database for up-to-date cancer treatment information. It is regularly updated and approved by cancer researchers. Have your doctor call the PDQ, or use your own FAX access.

For a 6-or-more-page FAX update about prostate cancer and its treatment options, call (301)402-5874. When instructed, enter the prostate cancer patient information code: 201229.

Wellness Community
2200 Colorado Ave.
Santa Monica, CA 90404-3504
(310) 453-2200

This is a growing network of programs for cancer patients and their families. Although concentrated in California, groups have sprung up in cities in the Deep South and East coast.

Appendix 2

Bibliography

The author owes a debt of gratitude to many experts, journals, authors and health care workers who were generous with their time and knowledge. A few of the works used as reference for this volume are listed below:

Bricklin, Mark., *The Practical Encyclopedia of Natural Healing: Revised Edition.*, New York, Penguin Books, 1990.

Cunningham, Chet., *The Prostate Problem.*, New York, Windsor-Pinnacle Books. 1990.

Dunn, Lavon J., *Nutrition Almanac,* Third Edition. New York, McGraw-Hill Publishing Co. 1990.

Editors, et.al., *Bircher-Benner Handbuch für Männer mit Prostataleiden.*, Bircher-Benner-Verlag GmbH, Bad Homburg, Germany. 1992.

Ethical Nutrients Corp., *Nutritional Research News,* issue 9.

Hoffman, Matthew and LeGro, William., *Disease Free: How to Prevent, Treat and Cure More Than 150 Illnesses and Conditions*. Pennsylvania; Rodale Press, 1993.

Hylton, William H., ed. *The Rodale Herb Book*. Emmaus, PA., Rodale Press, 1974.

Kordel, Lelord. *Natural Folk Remedies*. New York: G.P. Putnam's Sons, 1974.

Matsen, Jonn, M.D. *The Mysterious Cause of Illness: How to Overcome Every Disease from Constipation to Cancer* Canfield, Ohio, Fischer Publishing Co., 1988.

Merck Pharmaceutical Inc., *What Every Man Should Know About His Prostate* and *A Patient Guide: Proscar* ., Merck Pharmaceutical, Chapel Hill, NC., 1993.

Pschyrembel Klinisches Wörterbuch . DeGruyter, Berlin, Germany. 1986.

The Killer We Don't Discuss and *To Test or Not To Test:* articles in *Newsweek* magazine, volume cxxii, no.26, Dec. 27, 1993. pp 40-43.

Rossman, Isadore, M.D., *Looking Forward*., E.P. Dutton, 1989.

Rossman, Isadore, M.D., *The Best Treatment*., Bantam, 1992.

Rous, Stephen N., M.D., *The Prostate Book: Updated Edition*., *New York,* W.W. Norton, 1992.

Shapiro, Charles E., M.D. and Doheny, Kathleen. *The Well Informed Patient's Guide to Prostate Problems*. New York, Dell Publishing, 1993.

Simons, Anne, M.D., Hasselbring, Bobbie and Castleman, Michael., *Before You Call the Doctor.* New York, Fawcett Columbine, 1992.

Stoltz, Craig., *Prostate cancer: a bipartisan issue. USA weekend* magazine. Dec. 3-5 edition, 1993.

Treben, Maria. *Healing Through God's Pharmacy: Advice and Experiences With Medicinal Herbs.* Steyr, Austria, Wilhelm Ennsthaler, 1993.

Treben, Maria. *Maria Treben's Cures.* Steyr, Austria, Wilhelm Ennsthaler, 1980.

Index